THIRD EDITION

MOUNTAINEERING
FIRST AID

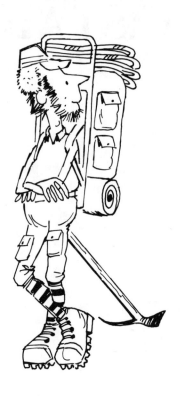

MOUNTAINEERING
FIRST AID

A GUIDE TO ACCIDENT RESPONSE AND FIRST AID CARE

THIRD EDITION

Martha J. Lentz, Ph.D., R.N.
Steven C. Macdonald, M.P.H., E.M.T.
Jan D. Carline, Ph.D.

Illustrations by Bruce Becker

The Mountaineers • Seattle

The Mountaineers: Organized 1906 "...to explore, study, preserve and enjoy the natural beauty of the Northwest..."

Copyright 1985 by The Mountaineers
All rights reserved

Published by The Mountaineers
306 Second Avenue West
Seattle, Washington 98119

Published simultaneously in Canada by Douglas & McIntyre Ltd.
1615 Venables Street, Vancouver, B.C. V5L 2H1

Edited by Sharon Bryan
Manufactured in the United States of America
First edition 1972
Second Edition 1975; second printing 1977, third printing 1978, fourth printing
    1979, fifth printing 1980, sixth printing 1983, seventh printing 1984
Third edition 1985

0 9
5 4 3

Library of Congress Cataloging in Publication Data

Lentz, Martha J.
    Mountaineering first aid.

    Rev. ed. of: Mountaineering first aid/Mitchell,
Dick. 2nd ed. 1975, c1972.
    Includes index.
    1. Mountaineering—Accidents and injuries.
2. First aid in illness and injury.   I. Macdonald,
Steven C.   II. Carline, Jan D.   III. Mitchell, Dick.
Mountaineering first aid.   IV. Title.
RC88.9.M6L46   1985   616.02'52   85-7115
ISBN 0-89886-092-X (pbk.)

CONTENTS

DEDICATION

Clint Kelley was a chairman of the Mountaineers First Aid Committee, an American Red Cross instructor trainer, and an important influence in the Mountaineering Oriented First Aid Program. Of all his many activities in mountaineering and conservation, he may have made his greatest contribution to the first aid program. Clint was a mentor to a whole generation of instructors, shaping their attitudes and approaches to first aid practice. Above all, he was a gentle and joyful instructor. This book is dedicated to the memory of Clint Kelley: leader, instructor, and good friend.

FOREWORD

In 1968, The Mountaineers, in cooperation with the Seattle-King County Chapter of the American Red Cross, developed a program of first aid instruction designed to meet the training requirements of those who ventured into the mountains where medical help was distant. It emphasized not only the specific first aid skills required in the event of an emergency but also the pre-trip preparation and response required at the scene of an accident should first aid or evacuation be necessary. Since its development, this program has seen a rapid growth in enrollment. The growth can be attributed to a tremendous effort by The Mountaineers in promoting first aid training, as well as a quality instructional program. This program is of benefit not only to the technical climber but any hiker who enjoys leisurely pursuits in unpopulated areas. It is hoped that by knowing first aid and the procedures to follow at the scene of an accident, many accidents will be prevented, and injuries reduced.

The Mountaineering Oriented First Aid (MOFA) course is built upon the Red Cross Standard First Aid and Personal Safety course. This course is taught in such a way as to give the student an opportunity to practice first aid skills using the supplies and materials that they carry into the field in their day pack. This cooperative training effort has been taught in the Seattle area for the past sixteen years and has met with continued student approval.

This, the third edition of, Mountaineering First Aid *is the effort of a number of instructors who have been teaching this program and felt a need to update the information presented and to adapt the Standard First Aid course to the particular needs of those who travel in the backcountry. Their efforts have produced this book, which can be used to enhance the first aid training taken by anyone who enjoys outdoor pursuits or participates in any type of mountain activity.*

NORMAN G. BOTTENBERG, Director
Safety Services
Seattle-King County Chapter
American Red Cross

ACKNOWLEDGMENTS

We would like to express our appreciation for the pioneering work of Dick Mitchell in mountaineering first aid. In addition to being one of the developers of the mountaineering first aid program in Seattle, he took the experience of that program and used it to produce the first two editions of *Mountaineering First Aid*. We have benefited not only from his work, but also from participating in the mountaineering first aid program. We would like to thank the students and instructors of that program, whose interest and enthusiasm have contributed to our thinking on mountaineering first aid.

Gordon Pfister, Ph.D., whose ideas and concerns have become an integral part of this manuscript, supplied a practical perspective, which included the actual rescue of an injured hiker. A project of this kind frequently requires a catalyst to bring people together and make a beginning; Mike Bryg, chairman of the Mountaineers First Aid Committee (1981–1984), was that catalyst.

Roger Andersen, Steve Bezruchka, M.D., Eric Larson, M.D., Ed Peters, Susan Price, M.D., and Jim Wilkerson, M.D., generously reviewed and provided suggestions for improvement of this manuscript. While we have used their ideas and suggestions, any errors are attributable only to the authors.

Finally, we would like to thank our spouses for their support and encouragement when we spent yet another evening or entire weekend working on this manuscript.

INTRODUCTION

When an injury occurs in the mountains, a first aider encounters a situation very different from that in a city. In the city, telephones, ambulances, and advanced medical help are only minutes away. In the mountains, getting to a phone may require hours of difficult travel. Getting outside help to the injured requires even more time, sometimes days. Rather than being responsible for the care of the injured person for a few minutes, the mountaineering first aider will need to provide care for hours or days.

The time needed to get the injured to medical care multiplies the responsibilities of the first aider. For example, contact lenses left in place on an unconscious victim will, after a number of hours, cause damage to the surface of the eyes. In the city, where the victim will quickly be taken to a hospital, eye care will be provided by the hospital's staff. In the mountains, the responsibility to detect and remove the contact lenses falls on the first aider.

The harsh mountain environment can pose a threat to healthy and strong persons, to say nothing of someone who has been injured or is ill. Exposure to heat, cold, high altitude, and inclement weather can cause problems infrequently encountered in the city. Keeping a victim warm is much more difficult on a snowy mountain slope than in a heated building. Storms, avalanches, and rockfall pose additional threats to the injured as well as to the first aider.

The problems of providing first aid in an extreme environment are made even more difficult by lack of equipment. All the first aider will have to work with is what the party has carried in with them or can be improvised. Selecting and packing equipment before leaving home must be done with the knowledge of some of the special problems associated with first aid in the mountains.

The first two editions of *Mountaineering First Aid* addressed the special problems of providing first aid in the mountains. This edition continues that emphasis. Changes have been made to bring the content up to date based on recent research, sections have been revised or expanded based on experience in the Mountaineering First Aid program and actual accident situations, and some entirely new material has been included.

Changes in format have been made as well. Important material has been highlighted by the use of numbers, bullets (marks to the left of text), and boxes. If actions need to be done in a specific order, they are numbered. If the actions do not need to be performed in a particular order, bullets have been used. Boxes have been used to summarize basic information and principles of first aid care.

This book provides basic information needed for first aid and prevention of illnesses in the mountains. Reading a book can provide information but does not offer an opportunity to practice skills nor the experiences from which to develop the judgment to use first aid skills wisely. Participation in a first aid course with plenty of opportunity to practice is a necessary step in developing skills. A first aid course will also provide the opportunity to practice making judgments about the best way to treat an injury before it must be done in a real accident situation. This book is NOT a substitute for a first aid course.

DEFINING FIRST AID:
CARING FOR THE PERSON WHO HAS BEEN HURT

First aid is defined as "the immediate care given to a person who has been injured or suddenly taken ill." To you, as a first aider, this means two very important things:

- That the first aid you perform must be IMMEDIATE. In some cases you should respond in less than a minute; in other cases you can wait minutes before doing something. But in nearly every problem encountered in the mountains, the first aid must be started in a relatively short time, even though evacuation may be delayed for hours or days.
- First aid is the immediate CARE given. This care includes not only bandaging or splinting the victim's physical injuries and protecting them from the environment, but also caring for the victim's entire mental and physical being. A wound is more than just bleeding. It involves pain, concern, anxiety, worry, and apprehension. All of these mental and emotional as well as physical needs must be attended to by the first aider.

Nearly all injured people want help. They want to know they will be all right; they want reassurance. This does not mean you should lie to them. It does mean they want the assurance of knowing someone qualified is there to help. They want to know what their injuries are (approximately) and what the first aider plans to do. In short, they usually want someone to talk to. This serves the first aider's needs too, since it enables him or her to determine how well the care given is working (does that make it hurt less?), and relieves the first aider's apprehension. This process, talking and attending to the victim's emotional needs, is called Tender Loving Care (TLC). It includes keeping the victim warm, comfortable, fed, busy, interested, happy, confident... and brave, and reverent, if applicable. TLC is extremely important, being one of the most effective actions a first aider can provide. TLC requires no special equipment; it is always available, even in remote areas, wherever there is a concerned rescuer. Its use cannot be overemphasized.

Chapter 1: Before Going into the Mountains

CAUSES AND PREVENTION OF INJURIES

For over thirty years, the American Alpine Club has been publishing the annual report of its Safety Committee as a booklet entitled *Accidents in North American Mountaineering*. It is a sobering account of serious injuries and sudden illnesses that befall mountaineers, with analyses of specific incidents and statistics on deaths, injuries, and causes. On average, thirty-five climbers are reported killed in the United States each year, with another hundred injured, not including skiing or hiking accidents.

There is a difference between accidents and injuries: an accident is an incident, or event; an injury involves harm to the body. The prevention of injuries includes consideration of both the causes of accidents and the causes of injuries.

Mountaineering injuries result from one of three circumstances: a climber falling (on rock or into a crevasse); something falling on a climber (rocks, avalanche); or the effects of some environmental extreme (such as cold or altitude). A variety of factors can cause accidents, ranging from judgmental error (such as exceeding one's abilities) to simple failure of equipment (although breakage of climbing hardware is currently quite rare). These factors can be called "contributory" causes: they often contribute to an accident, but they do not in themselves cause an injury. The injury results from a more immediate cause, such as a fall.

The following are examples of contributing causes from the American Alpine Club's *Accidents in North American Mountaineering*:

- *Equipment failure:*
    hardware breakage: piton, nut, ascender, etc.
- *Bad judgment using equipment:*
    climbing unroped
    using inadequate equipment: no hard hat, etc.
    failure of rappel
    placing no protection
    faulty use of crampons
- *Performance/judgment error:*
    exceeding abilities
    climbing alone
    loss of control on voluntary glissade
    failure to follow route
    party separated

• *Environmental conditions:*
  bad weather
  darkness

Perhaps the term "accident" is misleading. Mountaineering injuries are not accidental in the sense of being random or totally unpredictable. As the analyses from the Safety Committee show, the causes of an injury are readily apparent when the environmental conditions and the capabilities of the climber are known. The prevention of that injury involves assuring a reasonable match between the performance of the climber and the demands of the environment.

For example, when you are in an environment where there is a high risk of injury from rocks falling on your head, the use of a climbing helmet can prevent injury. The helmet will not stop the rocks from falling, but it can prevent the rock from hurting your head. Alternatively, you can choose a route that does not expose you to rockfall. Prevention, therefore, involves either altering an immediate cause of injury (rockfall), or altering a contributory cause (not using a helmet).

Risk and Safety

Rockfall is a risk of going into the mountains. But what is safe? *Risk* is a number, a statistic, which indicates the likelihood that an event will occur. For example, out of the 6000 people who try to climb Washington state's Mount Rainier each year, an average of three people die, so the odds of death are one in 2000. *Safety* is a judgment call, a decision about how much risk the climber is willing to accept. The decision to climb Mount Rainier may be made because he or she feels that the benefits, enjoyment, and a sense of accomplishment justify the risks. For some climbers, the sense of risk actually increases the benefit; i.e., the greater the risk, the better the experience, as far as they are concerned.

People vary in their willingness to take risks. An extremely cautious person maintains a large gap between his or her capabilities and the demands imposed by the environment—you could say a large "margin of safety." The extreme example is the person who stays home when the avalanche danger is low to moderate, rather than choosing a route along a ridge top. At the other end of the scale is the person who maintains a narrow gap between his or her capabilities and the task demands, a small "margin of safety." This would describe the person who pushes himself or herself near the point of exhaustion to bag just one more peak.

Acceptable Risk

How safe is "safe enough?" It would be impossible to totally eliminate risk from any part of society, let alone mountaineering. Further, willingness to take risks and challenge ourselves can be an important growth experience. The decision is to limit oneself to some "acceptable risk." The amount of risk that is acceptable for one person is not necessarily the same as that for the next person, as capabilities and desires differ. Recognizing those limits is the basis for prevention.

The limits themselves can be altered, as well. Capabilities can be improved, by training, physical conditioning, and experience. It is equally important to recognize that capabilities can be reduced, due to hypothermia, exhaustion, or inadequate oxygen. The individual can be protected, through the use of equipment such as ropes, hardhats, and ice axes. The environmental hazard can be reduced by doing a different route or waiting for better weather. Arriving at an acceptable level of risk involves maintaining an adequate margin of safety, and this requires the use of judgment.

Judgment

Judgment may mean deciding that a particular pitch requires a belay rope and the placing of protection. It may mean deciding that the summit attempt has to be postponed for today. In general, the person who routinely takes risks that exceed his or her abilities is probably "unsafe." Exceeding abilities may actually be the number one cause of mountaineering injuries.

The *Climbing Code* of The Mountaineers provides a guideline for safe practice. It includes:

- Carry at all times the clothing, food, and equipment necessary.
- Keep the party together and obey the leader or majority rule.
- Never climb beyond your ability and knowledge.
- Never let judgment be overruled by desire when choosing the route or turning back.

In summary, being aware of the causes of accidents will help you in preventing injuries. Both your enjoyment and your safety are best assured through setting a level of acceptable risk. Setting that level should be a conscious decision, based on sound judgment.

BEING PREPARED

A moment's thought about the mountaineering environment may make the need for advance preparation apparent. The mountains, rivers, deserts, and other areas of the wilderness do not care about people. They do not operate for our comfort or our safety. While we may think of them as beautiful or refreshing or challenging, the fact remains that they are physical features, much bigger and more powerful than we are.

It is too late to begin thinking about first aid response after an injury has occurred. Some preparation must take place before ever leaving town and some must occur during the trip itself. Such advance preparation assists both in preventing injuries and in assuring that when an injury does occur, the response will be rapid and effective.

Essentials of First Aid Response

MENTAL PREPARATION. In order to deal with the problem of an injury or sudden illness in this unsympathetic environment, you need to have a working knowledge of first aid. You must be able to organize a first aid response and apply it to the situation at hand. Adequate planning also includes: choosing a trip leader; discussing and selecting a route; checking predicted weather and trail conditions; reviewing the capability of the party members; and deciding what equipment and supplies should be taken.

PHYSICAL PREPARATION. Physical preparation involves both general physical fitness and conditioning, and the ability to perform hands-on first aid procedures. Reading a book about putting on a splint or giving CPR is a good start, but it is incomplete knowledge until the physical experience of actually doing it has been repeated often enough to master the skill.

GROUP PREPARATION. Before leaving the trailhead, party members need to be sure that they all agree on the route (especially if there are areas of possible confusion or high risk), and have divided up party equipment. The leader should identify members with first aid experience, as well as members with special medical or physical problems.

During the trip, ALL party members should think of possible evacuation routes, possible bivouac points, and more generally, what they would do if someone became sick, lost, or injured. That does not mean that one has to think of nothing else (that would make the trip dreary indeed), but all too often the opposite occurs and NO ONE ever thinks about these ugly possibilities. Every party member should periodically mentally rehearse "What would we do if...?"

MATERIAL PREPARATION. Material preparation includes the acquisition, testing, and organizing of the equipment and supplies needed for the trip. When packing for an outing, enough supplies must be included to sustain party members under the worst possible circumstances. Broken ankles or twisted knees have a nasty way of occurring where conditions are the worst in terms of weather and terrain. A prepared person can at least survive, even if he or she has some degree of discomfort. An unprepared one sometimes may not survive!

Each member of the group should ALWAYS assume that an emergency bivouac will be required and pack accordingly. This does not mean that everyone need carry a sleeping bag, a stove, and a tent. Each party member should, however, have enough equipment to survive the night under the worst conditions for that time of year and locality. If the trip will be limited to trail hiking in a low, forested, summer environment with a forty-eight-hour forecast of clear and mild weather, then emergency bivouac equipment might include only some extra food and clothing. The party could easily survive if an overnight stay were necessary. Note that the word is "survive," not "enjoy" the night. If the weather were to become wet or cold, then more than this minimal amount of equipment would be needed.

It is every individual's choice how much discomfort he or she is prepared to endure. (Of course, the party member who is always ill-prepared and must borrow from the others is usually not appreciated.) Not only must each member prepare for the worst when packing, but also prepare for the possible incident when care may need to be given to others. It is a responsibility of each party member to carry along a few additional items in excess of personal needs that could be given the victim of an injury or sudden illness. There is an interesting psychological reason for this. Often there is a tendency to withhold the donation of personal equipment to a victim, particularly under inclement weather conditions. It comes from a feeling (with good justification) that the donor will need it later. Therefore, each member MUST feel that there are articles in the pack in EXCESS of personal needs.

The Ten Essentials

A number of years ago, The Mountaineers came up with the idea of the "Ten Essentials." These are the basic things that EVERYONE should have on EVERY backcountry trip. They include:

- A map of the area
- A compass
- A flashlight with extra batteries and bulb
- Extra food
- Extra clothing, including raingear
- Sunglasses and sunscreen
- A pocketknife
- Matches in a waterproof container
- A candle or other firestarter
- A first aid kit

Five other pieces of equipment are strongly recommended—so strongly, in fact, that it really should be a list of the "fifteen essentials."

- *Full water bottle*. Your body loses water through evaporation while you hike, and it needs to be replaced. The assumption that there will be a little creek somewhere along the way is too often not true. Even more discouraging is the fact that more and more of our water, even in the backcountry, is not as pure as we would like. Take your water from home, and when a refill is needed, make sure the water is treated either through chemical means or by boiling.
- *Ground insulation*. (Roughly $12 \times 18 \times \frac{3}{8}$ inches). Loss of body heat, particularly during cold or wet weather, can be very rapid. If each member of the party carries a small piece of foam pad, a victim can easily be insulated from the ground or snow.

- *Tube shelter.* In the mountains, staying dry and out of the wind are the most important steps in staying warm. A tube shelter is an eight-foot tube of medium weight plastic that can readily be set up as a tent (complete with floor), a lean-to, or a windbreak.
- *Emergency blanket* (weight two ounces). These aluminized flexible mylar sheets reflect body heat extremely efficiently, preventing excess body heat loss. Roughly 60 by 80 inches when unfolded, they collapse to only 2 × 4 × ½ inches.
- *Signalling devices.* Whistles and mirrors make good signalling devices to attract attention. In particularly remote areas of wilderness, pocket flares or smoke grenades may be useful.

In special environments, such as on snow or glacier, additional equipment will be essential, including a shovel; a stove with fuel, a pan and cover; avalanche cord and/or a radio beacon (such as PIEPS or Skadi); and a rescue pulley.

None of these materials will do the slightest good if: one won't use them (I don't need light, I have eyes like a... CRUNCH! TUMBLE! SPLAT!); one doesn't know how to use them correctly (does the compass point to camp or away from camp?); or one didn't remember to bring them.

The Mountaineering First Aid Kit

Many people have a false sense of security with a first aid kit. A kit is not a magic device that cures all ills. Without the knowledge of what to use or when to use it, the items in a kit are useless. This can be especially true when using a commercially purchased prepackaged one. A competent first aider should be able to do a great number of first aid procedures with no more equipment than two bare hands and material normally found in any hiker's pack. The first aid kit contains a few additional specialized materials unique to first aid needs.

The kit should be small and compact, yet contain all the necessary materials. It should be light and easily packed, sturdy, and waterproof. A coated nylon stuff bag seems ideal until one wishes to get at something in the bottom. A plastic box with a tight lid makes a good container, but may not pack away as well as a bag. A metal box can be used, and in an emergency could be used to melt snow or warm water. But metal makes it heavier. Any first aid kit is a collection of compromises. Probably no two experts will pack exactly alike, and some will pack differently over time. There are dozens of commercial first aid kits on the market—many of which are barely adequate. There are also a number of different published lists of recommended contents. When selecting or assembling a first aid kit, consider the following general guidelines.

- Ensure that there is enough bulk to absorb a significant quantity of blood. In the backcountry, severely bleeding wounds are a common type of injury and sterile absorbent material cannot be readily improvised.

- Consider the area you are traveling into and pack accordingly. If traveling on glacier, for example, where there are no trees and ice axes cannot be spared, a wire ladder splint would be extremely valuable if a fracture occurs.

>   *Wire splints* are of two kinds. One is woven of a light weight wire. It can be purchased either prepackaged at some outdoor equipment stores or as "hardware cloth" at a hardware store. Its value is minimal for all but the smallest of fractures. The second type is made of much stiffer wire and is known as a "ladder splint." These are perhaps more difficult to obtain, but can be found through medical or ambulance supply outlets. The ladder splint is more versatile, useful for splinting virtually any fracture of the upper or lower extremities.

- Avoid carrying drugs. If you need something for your personal use, consult your family physician and let him or her explain its limitations, dangers, and directions for use. If you give medication to someone else, you are no longer practicing first aid, you are practicing medicine (without a license). What happens if the victim is that one person in 100,000 who is allergic to that particular drug? No matter how severe the pain or your need to "do something," it is very strongly recommended that you not share any form of medication.
- Carry first aid and rescue directions. Since no one's memory is perfect, carry a small booklet of information on what first aid to perform for various injuries or what rescue techniques should be initiated.
- Carry first aid report forms and a pencil. A first aid report form serves as a checklist to ensure that everything possible has been done for the victim and that those going for help have correct and accurate information. It allows you to collect the information while it is available and readily remembered. Trusting only to memory, you may inaccurately recall vital signs, injuries, times, locations, and so on.

With these thoughts in mind, the following specific items are recommended as guidelines:

Recommended Contents of First Aid Kit

ITEM	QUANTITY AND SIZE	USE
Bandaids	6 1-inch	minor wounds
Butterfly bandages	3, various sizes	minor lacerations
Sterile gauze pads	4 4 × 4-inch (roughly)	larger wounds
Carlisle "Battle" dressing (or sanitary napkin)	1 4-inch	severe bleeding
Nonadherent dressings	2 4 × 4-inch (roughly)	abrasions, burns
Roller gauze (or self-adherent roller bandage)	2 rolls, 2 inches × 5 yards	holding dressings on
Athletic tape	2-inch roll	multiple use
Triangular bandage	2	sling, cravat
Moleskin/molefoam	4 to 6 inches	blisters
Benzoin, tincture	½-ounce plastic bottle	adhesive, protects skin
Betadyne swabs (povidone iodine)	2 packages	antiseptic
Alcohol pads	3 packages	cleanse skin
Thermometer	30° C (90° F) to 41° C (105° F)	estimate body temperature
Sugar packets	2 packages	diabetes
Aspirin	6 tablets	headache, pain
Elastic bandage	1	sprains

Miscellaneous useful items may also include: safety pins, tweezers or needle for splinters, scissors, and several coins for a phone call.

Chapter 2: When an Injury Occurs

SEVEN STEPS FOR FIRST AID RESPONSE

When an accident occurs, many things need to be done. Some things must be done immediately, other things must wait until what has happened is better understood. The seven steps provide, in order of priority, an outline that can be followed in any accident situation. Each of the seven steps listed below will be discussed in detail in later sections.

STEP 1: TAKE CHARGE OF THE SITUATION. Objective: To get the party under control for maximum group response in a minimum of time. The designated leader must take charge of the situation immediately, organizing and assigning specific individuals to do certain tasks. If no leader has previously been agreed upon, then someone must become the self-appointed leader and assume these responsibilities. Other party members must become good followers.

STEP 2: APPROACH THE VICTIM SAFELY. Objective: To avoid further injury to the victim and keep other party members safe. Approach to the victim must be rapid but safe. It is important not only to protect the victim from further harm caused by rockfall, avalanche, or falling rescuers, but to protect the rest of the party as well.

STEP 3: PERFORM EMERGENCY RESCUE AND URGENT FIRST AID. Objective: To treat conditions that can cause loss of life within a few minutes. In a few instances, immediate rescue may be the most urgent care the first aider can provide. If the victim is in an area of high risk of snow or rock avalanche or extreme lightning danger, quickly move him or her to a safer location. Check, as a minimum, to see if the victim has stopped breathing, has no pulse, or is bleeding severely, and treat for these.

STEP 4: PROTECT THE VICTIM. Objective: To reduce the physical and emotional demands on the victim. Whatever the extent of the injuries, the victim will require protection from the environment, either hot or cold. Talk to the victim, explaining who you are and what you are doing and plan to do. TLC is important in reducing the emotional demands to which the victim must respond.

STEP 5: CHECK FOR OTHER INJURIES. Objective: To identify ALL injuries, major and minor. Once the life threatening emergencies have been identified and controlled, the victim can be examined in more detail. Be extremely thorough.

STEP 6: PLAN WHAT TO DO. Objective: To organize activities so that maximum treatment is provided with minimum cost to both the victim and the party. After urgently needed first aid has been given, initial protection from the environment has been provided, and all the victim's injuries have been identified, time should be spent planning what further tasks must be done. The leader must evaluate the victim's injuries, party size and physical condition, terrain, weather, and the party's location with respect to outside assistance. In short, the situation needs cool analysis and development of a comprehensive plan of action.

STEP 7: CARRY OUT THE PLAN. Objective: To accomplish treatment of the victim, and ensure the safety and well being of other party members. After a complete examination of the entire accident situation and development of a course of action, the party is ready to carry out its plans. If the plan is for self evacuation, guidance and continued observation of the victim will be needed to ensure his or her safety. If outside assistance is requested, the party should expect that in mountaineering situations it will take six to twenty-four hours for help to arrive. Changes in the victim's condition, or changes in terrain and weather, may require altering the plan of action.

STEP 1: TAKE CHARGE OF THE SITUATION

Taking charge is a matter of leadership. When someone is injured or is suddenly taken ill, a rapid response is often needed. These situations are upsetting to everyone involved. Even usually active and responsible persons may need guidance or directions to accomplish simple tasks. Thus, a strong leader is necessary to ensure that rapid and organized response occurs.

In well-planned parties, the leader of the group of people is clearly designated in advance. Often parties will designate a "first aid leader" as well. Even in small groups, in an injury situation a single leader is absolutely necessary. The immediate role of the leader is to take charge, assign tasks for people to do (in steps two through seven), and then to manage what goes on.

Leadership

The concept of leadership seems to many of us to be mystical or abstract. Leadership can be as simple as taking charge of the situation and then using your intuition to guide your decisions. It is more useful to think of leadership as "managing," a more concrete approach. Management of a scene involves doing the following:

- Be aware of all aspects of the situation.
- Try to avoid becoming so focused on one particular aspect of the problem that you lose the overall picture (remember the saying about "not seeing the forest for the trees"?).
- Observe and inquire.
- Seek out information and advice from other members of the party.

In a situation that is not an emergency, the usual leadership style is consensus, where all party members agree on a course of action. In an emergency situation, this is not efficient, and a leader needs to decide on some action quickly. The essence of step one is simply to take charge and to be sure that steps two, three, four, and so on, are done.

Taking Charge

There are a number of ways of taking charge. The easiest is when you have been appointed "first aid leader" for a particular trip. Often, however, there is no appointed leader, and when a situation occurs everyone hesitates, waiting for someone else to do something. In that situation you have three choices: (1) offer; (2) assume leadership, stating the need for action; or (3) act—take the role by initiating action.

Once you have taken charge, there are different levels of management, each appropriate to different situations. When other members of the party have no idea what to do (possibly because, unlike you, they have not taken a first aid course), assigning tasks directly may work best. If they all know what to do, allowing tasks to be done by those who step in to do them may work well.

TASKS. No matter what type of leadership structure exists, there are certain tasks that must be accomplished in every mountaineering first aid situation. These tasks are unvarying, in that they will always need to be done. What can and will vary is how they will be accomplished. In a large party, the first aid leader will be able to delegate the tasks to a number of different people; in a small party, one person may have two or more tasks. The tasks are:

- Performing hands-on care: head-to-toe exam and first aid treatment
- Recording findings
- Monitoring the victim: ever-present contact, staying with the victim constantly, listening and providing reassurance
- Inventorying equipment
- Scouting the area: for hazards, other victims, and so on
- Going for help (when necessary)

Followership

Other party members must be good followers, assuming responsibility for their assigned tasks willingly and providing the leader with information about what they have accomplished or difficulties encountered. For example, in a hypothetical situation with two victims and five rescuers, the leader would talk with the two victim examiners (a "leader's conference") after about ten minutes, in order to size up the situation, while the other two people stay with the victims. The wisdom of any leader's decisions is determined by the quality of the information given by the followers.

In summary, step one of the seven steps for first aid response is to take charge: assign tasks to people and then go on to step two.

STEP 2: APPROACH THE VICTIM SAFELY

Approach to the victim must be rapid but safe. Do not approach from directly above if there is a possibility of rock or snow slide. Approach should be from the side or even below, if possible. It is important to protect not only the victim, but the rest of the party as well, from further harm from rockfall, avalanche, or falling rescuers.

If the terrain is steep, difficult, or hazardous, keep the rest of the party back as one or two of the best qualified people approach the victim. Have the others begin to scout the area, inventory equipment, prepare a shelter, and so on, as necessary.

Those who are approaching the victim should be prepared with the proper equipment, particularly if the victim is perched precariously on a ledge or in an otherwise difficult position. This equipment might include slings, carabiners, rope, insulation, clothing, and first aid kits. Additionally, those rescuers should not put themselves in jeopardy by neglecting the usual precautions, such as placing protection and remaining attached to the rope in technical climbing situations.

Another aspect of approaching safely arises when the victim has been attacked by a bear or other wild animal, or bitten by a snake. Ask yourself: Where is the animal? Are you *sure* that snake is dead?

This book stresses preventing further injury, and the key to approaching the victim safely is the awareness that sometimes lightning does strike twice, so to speak. Rockfall often occurs twice in the same gully. Snow slides often occur one right after the other.

In summary, approach the victim rapidly but safely. Protect the victim, and the rest of the party, from the possibility of further injuries.

STEP 3: PERFORM EMERGENCY RESCUE AND URGENT FIRST AID

There are several situations which require immediate action to prevent further injury to or death of the victim and/or injury to the first aiders. After approaching the victim safely, an INITIAL RAPID CHECK must be made to determine if any of these situations exist:

1. *Environmental hazards.* Look around you: does the environment expose you to rockfall, avalanche, or other dangers?
2. *Absence of breath or pulse.* Speak to the victim: If the victim can respond verbally, you know he or she is able to breathe. If the victim doesn't respond, check for breathing and pulse.
3. *Severe bleeding.* Look at victim from head to toe, look under clothing, look under the victim: Is blood pooled underneath, being absorbed by clothing, or is blood being held inside rain gear?

These actions need to be done in a few moments if they are to be successful.

Environmental Hazard

Rockfall, avalanche, lightning, and other environmental hazards may pose an immediate threat to victims and rescuers. These hazards may necessitate moving the victim as rapidly as possible. The leader must weigh the danger posed by the environment against the potential for harm to the victim from a hasty move. The leader must also determine the type of transfer that is best for the victim and keep the number of party members exposed to the hazard at a minimum.

When moving the victim, support the head, neck, and back. Keep the victim's entire body in a straight line and avoid any twisting movement. A person can be dragged to safety by grasping his or her clothing near the shoulders, supporting the head on the rescuer's forearms, and pulling in a straight line.

Absence of Breath or Pulse

Absence of breathing or pulse may result in death after only a few minutes. Cessation of breathing or difficult breathing may be caused by: lightning; crushing or suffocation by ice blocks, snow, or rock; choking or strangulation by rope, clothing, or pack straps; falls or blows on the head; drowning; inadequate ventilation during cooking in snow caves or tents; or puncture wounds of the chest. Whatever the cause, unless immediate action is taken, the victim will most likely die within a few minutes. Removing the cause, as in strangulation, or removing the victim from the hazard, as with inadequate ventilation when cooking, may be all that is needed to restore breathing. If the problem is a puncture wound to the chest, seal the wound off immediately, first with your hand then with an airtight dressing. If breathing has stopped, start mouth-to-mouth artificial respiration.

When there is no pulse present, CPR (cardiopulmonary resuscitation) is needed. The procedures for effective and safe CPR are beyond the scope of this book, requiring practice on special mannequins. CPR procedures are NEVER practiced on another person. Taking a class in CPR procedures is highly recommended.

Checking for Absence of Breath and Pulse

1. **CHECK FOR RESPONSIVENESS.** Speak loudly to the victim, tap his or her shoulder lightly: if the victim is not responsive, then open the airway.
2. **OPEN AIRWAY.** When there is NO reason to suspect a neck or back injury, place the palm of one hand on his or her forehead, and tilt the victim's head back. Place the tips of the fingers of the other hand under the bony part of the victim's chin, and lift the jaw up and forward.

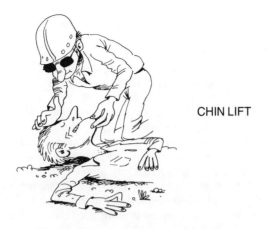

CHIN LIFT

When there IS reason to suspect a neck or back injury, use the jaw thrust method. Place your hands on each side of the victim's head, and push on the base of the jaw to push the jaw up and forward. DO NOT tilt the head back.

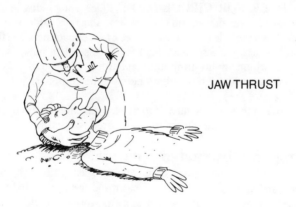

JAW THRUST

3. **CHECK FOR BREATHING.** With your head turned so you can see the victim's chest and abdomen, place your ear and cheek next to the victim's nose and mouth.

   - LOOK for movement of the chest and abdomen.
   - LISTEN for the sound of air movement.
   - FEEL for air movement against the side of your cheek.
   - If you see chest and abdomen movement without hearing or feeling air movement, the victim is trying to breathe, but the airway is still obstructed. Recheck position of the head and jaw to make sure the airway is open.

- IF THE VICTIM IS NOT BREATHING, give four quick breaths:

  A. Pinch the victim's nose closed between your thumb and forefinger while maintaining the head tilt with palm pressure on the forehead. When using the jaw thrust, seal the nose with the side of your cheek.

  B. Take a deep breath, open your mouth wide, and make a tight seal over the victim's mouth.

  C. Breathe into the victim's mouth two times. As you breathe into the mouth, watch for the victim's chest to rise. Be sure to look up and take a deep breath, to completely refill your lungs between breaths. Each breath should last one to one and a half seconds, to allow adequate time for good chest expansion. If you are unable to blow air into the victim's lungs, the airway may be obstructed. Reposition the victim's head and try again. If you are still unable to blow air into the victim's lungs, use the *procedures for clearing an obstructed airway,* described in a later section.

4. **CHECK FOR CIRCULATION.** Place your index and middle fingers on the victim's voice box and then slide your fingers down the side of the victim's neck to the space between the voice box and neck muscle. Feel for a pulse. If a pulse is present, continue mouth-to-mouth breathing. If the pulse is absent, mouth-to-mouth breathing needs to be combined with CPR.

Continue through these procedures step by step until the victim is breathing on his or her own, or until you are too exhausted to continue.

Clearing an Obstructed Airway

If the victim is conscious but unable to speak, or if the victim is unconscious and you have opened the airway and tried but failed to be able to give two breaths, the following steps are performed until the airway is cleared.

1. Give four abdominal thrusts. If the victim is *conscious,* stand behind him or her, circling the upper abdomen, slightly above the navel, with your arms. Grasp one of your fists with the other hand, with the thumb side placed against the middle of the abdomen, and give quick backward thrusts. If the victim is *unconscious,* position the victim on his or her back. Kneel astride the victim, place

the heel of one hand in the middle of the victim's abdomen slightly above the navel, place the heel of the other hand over it, and give quick upward thrusts.

2. Check for any foreign body in the mouth of an unconscious person. Slide a crooked finger along the inside of the victim's cheek, then sweep across the back of the mouth and bring out any obstructing objects.

3. Repeat attempts to give two breaths to the unconscious person.

The above steps are repeated in rapid sequence until successful in clearing the airway. If the victim does not begin breathing when the obstruction has been cleared from the airway, begin mouth-to-mouth breathing.

Severe Bleeding

Major wounds can cause severe, life-threatening bleeding. Since severe bleeding can be fatal in minutes, quick, decisive action is mandatory. The victim must have a rapid head-to-toe exam, which can be completed in only a few moments. Look to see if there are any obvious signs of severe bleeding. Arterial bleeding occurs in pulses or spurts of bright red blood. Venous bleeding is dark red and flows smoothly, without spurting. Check to see if blood is pooling under the victim, or is being absorbed into heavy clothing or being held inside rain clothes. If severe bleeding is encountered, treatment must be started immediately. Don't wait to take off your pack to get out a sterile dressing. The following steps should be taken to control any major bleeding:

1. Immediately apply DIRECT PRESSURE to the bleeding area. DO NOT allow severe bleeding to continue while rummaging through packs for sterile dressings—use your bare hand if necessary. When a sterile dressing is available, place it directly over the wound. If the dressing becomes soaked with blood, place additional dressings on top of the old ones and continue to apply direct pressure. This stops the bleeding in nearly all instances. When you need your hand to do something else, you can replace manual pressure with a pressure dressing (compression dressing), as described in Chapter 3.

2. If the wound is on a limb, ELEVATE the bleeding extremity. Elevation reduces the blood pressure in a limb slightly and will slow bleeding. If there is an obvious fracture (broken bone) in the extremity, then elevating the limb is inadvisable. Fortunately, most bleeding is controllable by direct pressure alone.

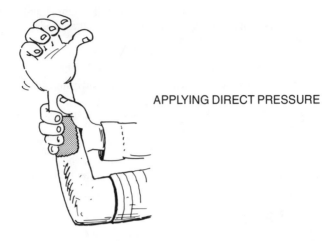

APPLYING DIRECT PRESSURE

3. Use PRESSURE POINTS. Anywhere that an artery can be felt pulsing as it passes over a bone is a potential pressure point. Compression at this point will reduce the flow of blood through the artery. In general, pressure points are only useful until a pressure dressing is in place.
4. If these measures fail, and the wound is on a limb, and *only if the bleeding continues to be severe and life threatening,* apply a tourniquet. Apply it tightly enough to stop the bleeding, and once the tourniquet is in place, leave it on—DO NOT loosen it. Loosening can restart the bleeding and release toxins into the bloodstream. Tag or otherwise mark the victim to alert medical personnel that a tourniquet has been placed, and indicate the time of placement. Many physicians believe that the use of a tourniquet is *practically never justified.* The DECISION TO APPLY A TOURNIQUET IS ESSENTIALLY A DECISION TO SACRIFICE THAT LIMB TO SAVE THE LIFE.

When someone is bleeding, the amount of blood and the length of time needed to stop the bleeding tend to become distorted. Do not become discouraged; continue the efforts to stop the bleeding until successful.

In summary, the points of concern in step three are:
- To remove the victim and rescuers from environmental dangers
- To establish the victim's airway, breathing, and pulse
- To stop life-threatening bleeding

STEP 4: PROTECT THE VICTIM

Once urgently needed first aid has been completed, the victim immediately must be protected from the stresses of heat or cold, further injury, and unnecessary fear and worry. When a person is injured, unusual amounts of energy are needed to maintain normal body functions. Exposure to heat or cold places additional demands on the body which it may not be able to meet. These demands must be minimized. Even in mild weather, the victim may be losing heat. It is much easier to keep a victim warm than it is to rewarm a cold victim. The victim's head and trunk should quickly be covered with extra clothing to prevent heat loss. Protection from rain and snow is essential, as wetness can quickly drain away warmth. Use the victim's clothing before your own. Insulation can be placed under a cold victim by sliding pieces of clothing or strips of padding under limbs or in depressions in the ground. If the victim is too warm, loosen clothing and create shade with a tarp erected over the victim.

Initial protection from the elements can be done quickly and without moving the victim. Movement must wait until the complete check for further injuries has been finished and a treatment plan devised. An unconscious victim of trauma must be assumed to have sustained an injury to the back or neck, and should NOT be moved.

Some conditions may require that movement takes place before the finish of the complete check for injuries. Emergency rescue will require immediate movement, as will the need to perform CPR and, in some cases, artificial respiration. A victim experiencing severe hypothermia or shock will need to be moved quickly onto insulation to prevent heat loss that could quickly result in death.

A careless step on the victim's hand or the fall of a pack on an injured leg can quickly worsen the victim's condition. Keep additional rescuers away from the victim unless they are needed for the immediate care of the victim. Packs or other gear should be left at the edge of the accident area to prevent rescuers from tripping over a pack and falling on the victim. Care should be taken not to walk over the victim or to pass equipment over the victim that might be dropped.

Stresses of fear and worry can only add to the victim's discomfort. One rescuer should be designated to communicate with the victim. A victim wants someone to talk to, but will become confused and more anxious if several people are shouting all at the same time. Talking, attending to the victim's emotional needs (TLC), and explaining what will be done will convey a sense of caring and first aid competence. It is important to talk to an apparently unconscious victim, since he or she very well may hear you and be reassured. The early establishment of a calm and caring relationship will do much to reduce the stresses of the injury.

In summary, step four includes protecting the victim from the stresses of heat or cold, further injury, and unnecessary fear and worry.

STEP 5: CHECK FOR OTHER INJURIES

Victim assessment begins with the initial observation of the accident scene, and continues with the initial rapid check, full examination, and follow-up examinations of the victim. The intent of the assessment is to:

- Identify the victim's injuries, and the circumstances and events contributing to the victim's condition.
- Monitor the victim's condition until rescue is completed, so that any changes in the victim's condition can be taken into consideration.
- Provide information to rescuers and medical personnel about the nature of the victim's condition. Appropriate plans for evacuation will depend on this information.

Initial Observations

Information about the victim's condition can be gained by noting the circumstances of the accident. A long fall will probably result in greater injury than a short tumble. A fall onto rock should raise suspicion of a neck or back injury. Wet, cool weather should suggest hypothermia. Quickly observing these facts can help in estimating the type and severity of injury sustained by the victim. A victim having a minor injury such as a stubbed toe may not need to undergo a complete examination. In contrast, some victims may not be aware of their own serious injuries. Keep a high level of suspicion of the seriousness of any injury, particularly if you did not witness the accident.

When you arrive at the accident scene, introduce yourself to the victim. Give your name and an indication of your first aid training. Ask the victim if you may help. The victim has the right to refuse any aid. Additional explanation may help the victim to accept aid. Tell the victim what you are about to do. Even an apparently unconscious victim may be able to hear what you are saying, and may be calmed by knowing what to expect.

Ask the victim: What happened? How did it happen? When did it happen? What hurts? Do you have any other problems? Medical conditions? Allergies? Are you cold, hungry, or exhausted?

Information gained from a conscious victim is important in the identification of first aid needs. A victim who later becomes unconscious will not be able to answer questions. Ask similar questions of others who saw the accident or know the victim.

As you talk to the victim, observe: Is there any obvious deformity? Does the victim seem abnormally pale, sweaty, or nervous? Is the victim aware of the surroundings and able to respond reasonably to questions? Does the victim's position such as holding onto a broken elbow or forearm indicate the mechanism or type of injury? After these initial steps in assessment have been completed, the full victim examination may begin.

General Principles of Physical Examination

There are several principles that should guide the examination:

- **DO NO FURTHER HARM.** A gentle but firm touch should be used. A light brush of the hand will NOT be sufficient to discover injury.
- **BE COMPLETE AND SYSTEMATIC.** Examine every portion of the victim. Time is usually not a significant factor in proceeding with the examination. Do not be led astray by the obvious injury.
- **USE DIRECT OBSERVATION.** Rely on senses of vision, hearing, touch, and smell. Assume that there is an injury to a body part until you have directly observed otherwise. Get to bare skin, protecting the victim with a tarp or by quickly replacing clothing as one area of the body has been examined. Clothing may need to be cut to observe the skin. Cut the clothing so that it can be easily folded or taped together to retain its insulative value to protect the victim.
- **COMPARE BODY PARTS.** Some fractures or dislocations may be indicated only by an unusual shortening of a limb. Compare one limb with another, or with a rescuer's limb, to see if a deformity or unusual movement is present.
- **HAVE ONE PERSON DO THE EXAMINATION.** More than one set of hands on a victim at the same time may result in misleading findings, in addition to increasing the victim's anxiety.
- **MAKE MULTIPLE OBSERVATIONS.** Changes in a victim's condition can provide important information about injury when described to medical personnel, and may lead to changes in plans for first aid in the field.
- **RECORD ALL YOUR FINDINGS.** Use a second first aider to act as a recorder. Record the time as well as the finding itself.
- **RECORD BOTH SIGNS AND SYMPTOMS.** Signs are observable indications of illness, such as bleeding or deformity. Symptoms are the sensations reported by the victim, such as nausea or fatigue.

During the examination:

- Do not give first aid other than that needed to treat urgent problems. Treatment should wait until the full examination is completed and all injuries have been identified.
- Do not move the victim. A physical examination can be completed on a victim who is in a position other than flat on his or her back.
- Observe the victim's right to privacy when removing clothing. While it is essential to actually observe skin, the whole trunk need not be exposed while only a portion is being examined.

Head-To-Toe Examination

The head-to-toe is the systematic method of assuring that every portion of the victim's body is examined, so that no injury goes undiscovered. Specific indications of injury include:

- Deformity, such as abnormal length or shape of a body part
- Bruising or other discoloration
- Bleeding or other loss of fluids
- Swelling
- Abnormal movement of a body part, such as a joint moving in an abnormal direction
- Inability to move or limited range of motion
- Lack of expected symmetry, either in appearance or function
- Pain responses: generalized pain in an area, pain at a specific point, pain on motion, pain on touch (tenderness)

Ask the conscious victim about pain or sensation in each part of the body. Ask the victim to describe the pain: is it constant or intermittent, dull or sharp, getting better or worse? After you have asked the victim about sensation in the body part to be examined, look at the part, then touch the part, and only then ask the victim to move the part.

The unconscious victim may react in some way when called by name. Even if unable to respond to a verbal command, the victim may react to a painful stimulus such as a pinch on the ear lobe or deep pressure at the base of the thumbnail. The reaction may be a moan or a movement away from the painful stimulus. Medical conditions or allergies may be indicated by tags on bracelets or necklaces, or found on identification cards.

Proceed with the head-to-toe examination in the following steps.

1. Check the head: face, eyes, nose, mouth, ears, and scalp.
   - Look for signs of bleeding or presence of other fluid.
   - Look for any asymmetry in the face or in facial movements.
   - Look for any sign of fracture or other deformity.
   - Look in the ears for fluid.
   - Look for blood in the eye, or the presence of contact lenses. A contact lens can be seen by opening the lids and shining a light from the outer edge across the eye. The edge of the contact lens will be seen as the light bends across it.
   - Look in the victim's mouth for wounds or other injury (ask the victim to open his or her mouth).
   - Feel for any bumps, depressions, or blood. Start at the back of the head and work to the top and front of the head.
   - Have the victim follow your finger with his or her eyes, as you move your finger from side to side and up and down. Note any inability to move the eye. Both eyes should move at the same time in the same direction.

- DO NOT MOVE THE HEAD in the process of examination.
2. Check the neck, spine, and upper back.
   - Look for any obvious deformity or bleeding along the neck, including abnormal position of the head with respect to the neck.
   - Feel along the spine and upper back, beginning at the top of the neck. Feel for any indication of deformity, bleeding, tenderness, or muscular spasm.
   - DO NOT MOVE THE SPINE.
3. Check the chest and shoulders.
   - Look for any obvious deformity or discoloration.
   - Look for any indication of wounds or bleeding.
   - Look for any abnormal motion, such as one section of the chest collapsing while the rest expands.
   - Feel for pain or deformity over the upper shoulders and chest. Gentle pressure should be exerted on the ribs from side to side and from front to back, while noting any pain response.
   - Listen for any abnormal sounds on respiration or for the grating sounds of broken ribs.
4. Check the abdomen and lower back.
   - Look for any obvious deformity or discoloration.
   - Look for any indication of wounds or bleeding.
   - Feel the abdomen for any indication of muscle spasm or unusually tender areas.
   - Feel along the spine and lower back for any indication of deformity, bleeding, tenderness, or muscular spasm.
5. Check the pelvic area.
   - Look for obvious deformity or discoloration.
   - Look for any indication of wounds or bleeding.
   - Look for abnormal position of the leg. Rolling outward, for example, may indicate injury to the hip.
   - Feel for injury of the pelvic bones by pressing firmly from side to side, and pushing from front to back, noting any instability or pain response.
6. Check the buttocks.
   - Look for obvious swelling or discoloration.
   - Feel for irregularities or bleeding.
7. Check upper and lower extremities.
   - Look for obvious deformity or discoloration.
   - Look for any indication of wounds or bleeding.
   - Look for abnormal movement or position of the limbs.
   - Look for lack of symmetry between limbs.
   - Feel for tenderness, deformity.
   - Have the victim grip or push against your hand with his or her hand (DO THIS ONLY if no fracture is present). Compare

> the strength of response on one side with that on the other.
> - Have the victim push or pull against your hand with his or her foot (DO THIS ONLY if no fracture is present). Compare the strength of response on one side with that on the other.
> - Check the pulse above and below the site of any injury to determine if blood is flowing beyond the injury.

Vital Signs

Vital signs indicate the level of the body's vital functioning. Checking vital signs is an essential part of an examination. They may be measured in a separate step or may be done as part of the head-to-toe. These signs include pulse, breathing, skin color and temperature, pupillary reactions, state of consciousness, the sensation of pain, and ability to move. Normal values for the vital signs are given in the following box:

VITAL SIGNS	NORMAL VALUES
• Pulse	• 60–80/minute in adults, 80–100/minute in children, increased by exercise or fear, may be lower in athletes
• Breathing	• 12–15 breaths/minute in adults, 20–30 breaths/minute in young children
• Skin	• Underlying reddish tone; warm and dry to the touch
• Pupils of the eyes	• Regular in outline and the same size; contract upon exposure to light
• State of consciousness	• Fully alert, responsive to verbal and/or physical stimuli; aware of time, place, and location
• Sensation of pain and ability to move	• Reacts to stimuli and moves easily upon command

PULSE. The pulse indicates the rate at which the heart is pumping blood. The pulse can be felt at the wrist, in a hollow just back from the thumb. It may also be felt at the neck, just to the side of the Adam's apple. Note the pulse by using the first two fingers of the hand (not the thumb); count the number of beats in fifteen seconds and multiply by four. Also note the strength and regularity of the pulse. Record the findings and the time.

BREATHING. Rate and depth of breathing is an indication of how adequately the body is being supplied with oxygen. The difficulty or ease of breathing, its regularity, and any noises associated with breathing should be noted. Check the rate of breathing by placing a hand where the victim's chest and abdomen meet, counting the number of movements in a minute. Record the findings and the time. The presence of gurgling sounds or sputum coming from the mouth or nose should be also noted.

SKIN. The skin normally has an underlying reddish tone. Absence of this tone may be seen as ashen or pale color in Caucasians, dull ashen gray in black pigmented persons, and a dull yellowish brown in brown pigmented persons. The skin may also appear mottled, yellowish, bluish, or pale and white. The presence of sweat and any unusual warmth or coolness should be noted.

PUPILS OF THE EYE. Pupil response is an indication of central nervous system functioning. Unevenness in the size of the pupils, or slow reaction of the pupils to light, may indicate serious injury to the head. Pupil response may be checked by shading the eyes with a hand, then exposing the eyes to sunlight, or by flashing a light in the eyes. Both pupils should contract promptly and evenly. Note any differences between the eyes.

STATE OF CONSCIOUSNESS. The victim's state of consciousness is another indication of central nervous system functioning. Any departure from normal alertness should be noted, such as combativeness or confusion. The quality of speech—clear to slurred—may be an important sign of injury. If a victim seems unconscious, can he or she be awakened by verbal or painful stimuli?

PAIN AND MOVEMENT. Lack of reaction to painful stimuli may denote damage to the nervous system. Even an unconscious victim will move away from painful stimuli if there is no paralysis of the appropriate muscles. When testing for sensation, be careful not to give cues to the victim. Ask a conscious victim, "What am I touching?" rather than, "Can you feel this on your right leg?" An anxious victim, hoping not to be injured, may report feeling the touch. Movement should be accomplished easily upon command. Testing for the ability to move should begin with small movements, such as wiggling the fingers or toes. Then progress to larger movements, such as grasping with the hand or pushing with the foot. The last to be tested should be movements of the full limb. If you suspect a fracture, do not request the victim to move that limb. Similarly, do not request a victim with a suspected back or neck injury to sit up or move about.

RECORDING VITAL SIGNS. All vital signs should be recorded periodically. In the severely injured victim, vital signs should be taken every ten to fifteen minutes. In a victim with a minor injury, frequent taking of vital signs may not be necessary. Any worsening of the vital signs signals the first aider to repeat examination of the victim. Injuries that might have been missed or have gotten worse need to be identified, and the first aid plan altered.

The major components of checking for other injury are:

- **INITIAL OBSERVATIONS.** Note the circumstances of the injury and the initial appearance of the victim; introduce yourself to the victim
- **HEAD-TO-TOE EXAMINATION.** A systematic examination of the victim's body must be undertaken so that no injury goes undiscovered
- **VITAL SIGNS.** Repeated taking of the vital signs is an essential part of monitoring the victim's condition

The First Aid Report Form

The complete check for injury provides information on which to plan first aid, and for the decisions of medical personnel who will receive the severely injured victim. This information must be recorded if it is to be helpful. A first aider's ability to remember details is usually lessened by the stress and chaos of an accident scene. Information about the victim not recorded and forgotten is useless. Recorded information is needed by both those who are staying with the victim and those party members going out for help. Complete information must also accompany the victim when he or she is evacuated. The First Aid Report Form is designed to help the first aider accurately collect and record information.

There are three sections to the form: Start Here to record findings of the head-to-toe examination; the Vital Sign Record to note results of repeated observations; and the Rescue Request to be carried when going out for help.

START HERE. Begin with Start Here—where else? This section guides you through the head-to-toe examination. Record findings in the indicated places on the form, and note each step of first aid in the column to the right of findings. Findings not recorded immediately will likely be forgotten. Be sure to note the time of the examination.

VITAL SIGN RECORD. On the back of the Start Here section is space for recording repeated vital sign observations. Possible terms to describe the vital signs are suggested. Changes in the victim's condition over time may be noticed only if careful records are kept. Any improvement or deterioration in the vital signs may cause a change in first aid plans.

RESCUE REQUEST. Separate the completed Rescue Request and send it out if party members go for help. List what happened, what injuries were sustained, and the first aid given. On the back of the sheet, clearly describe the party's location and its plan. The party's resources should be included, as well as the type of assistance needed.

The details of Step 6 and Step 7 are described in Chapter 5, "Making a Plan and Carrying It Out." Chapter 3 discusses injuries to specific portions of the body and specific first aid actions that will be needed to make and carry out the plan.

© The Mountaineers

FIRST AID REPORT FORM

START HERE	FINDINGS	FIRST AID GIVEN

AIRWAY, BREATHING, CIRCULATION

INITIAL RAPID CHECK
(Chest Wounds, Severe Bleeding)

ASK WHAT HAPPENED:

ASK WHERE IT HURTS:

TAKE PULSE & RESPIRATIONS | PULSE | RESPIRATIONS

HEAD-TO-TOE EXAMINATION

HEAD: Scalp — Wounds
Ears, Nose — Fluid
Eyes — Pupils
Jaw — Stability
Mouth — Wounds

NECK: Wounds, Deformity

CHEST: Movement, Symmetry

ABDOMEN: Wounds, Rigidity

PELVIS: Stability

EXTREMITIES: Wounds, Deformity
Sensation & Movement
Pulses Below Injury

BACK: Wounds, Deformity

SKIN: Color
Temperature
Moistness

STATE OF CONSCIOUSNESS

PAIN (Location)

LOOK FOR MEDICAL ID TAG

ALLERGIES

VICTIM'S NAME | AGE

COMPLETED BY | DATE | TIME

TEAR HERE – KEEP THIS SECTION WITH VICTIM

DETACH HERE – SEND OUT WITH REQUEST FOR AID

RESCUE REQUEST

Fill Out One Form Per Victim

TIME OF INCIDENT		
AM	PM	DATE

NATURE OF INCIDENT
FALL ON: ☐ ROCK ☐ SNOW ☐ FALLING ROCK
☐ CREVASSE ☐ AVALANCHE
☐ ILLNESS ☐ EXCESSIVE ☐ HEAT ☐ COLD

BRIEF DESCRIPTION OF INCIDENT

INJURIES
(List Most Severe First)

PAIN (Location):

STATE OF CONSCIOUSNESS:

SKIN TEMP/COLOR:

FIRST AID GIVEN

RECORD:

	INITIAL		WHEN LEAVE SCENE
Time			
Pulse			
Respiration			

VICTIM'S NAME | AGE

ADDRESS

NOTIFY (Name) | RELATIONSHIP | PHONE

VITAL SIGN RECORD

Record TIME	BREATHS		PULSE		PULSES BELOW INJURY	PUPILS	SKIN	STATE OF CONSCIOUS-NESS	OTHER
	Rate	Character	Rate	Character					
		Deep, Shallow, Noisy, Labored		Strong, Weak, Regular, Irregular	Strong Weak Absent	Equal Size, React To Light, Round	Color Tempera-ture Moistness	Alert, Confused, Unresponsive	Pain, Anxiety, Thirst, Etc.

TEAR HERE – KEEP THIS SECTION WITH THE VICTIM

DETACH HERE – SEND OUT WITH REQUEST FOR AID

SIDE 2 RESCUE REQUEST

EXACT LOCATION (Include Marked Map If Possible)

QUADRANGLE: _____ SECTION: _____

AREA DESCRIPTION: _____

TERRAIN: ☐ GLACIER ☐ SNOW ☐ ROCK
☐ BRUSH ☐ TIMBER ☐ TRAIL
☐ FLAT ☐ MODERATE ☐ STEEP

ON SITE PLANS:
☐ Will Stay Put
☐ Will Evacuate To
Can Stay Overnight Safely ☐ Yes ☐ No
On Site Equipment: ☐ Tent ☐ Stove ☐ Food
☐ Ground Insulation ☐ Flare ☐ CB Radio

LOCAL WEATHER

EVACUATION: ☐ Carry-Out ☐ Helicopter
☐ Lowering ☐ Raising

EQUIPMENT: ☐ Rigid Litter
☐ Food ☐ Water ☐ Other

PARTY MEMBERS REMAINING:
Beginners _____ Intermediate _____ Experienced

NAME _____ NOTIFY (Name) _____ PHONE _____

NOTIFY:
IN NATIONAL PARK: Ranger
OUTSIDE NATIONAL PARK: Sheriff/County Police.
RCMP (Canada)

Chapter 3: First Aid for Specific Conditions

INJURIES

Wounds

In mountaineering, wounds occur in a number of ways: from rockfall or falls on rock; from improper use of an ice ax, crampons, or knife; from explosion of a gas stove, and so on. The cause will determine the type of wound: a slip and slide on steep rock can cause abrasions; a mistake with a sharp knife can cause a laceration; stepping on someone in your crampons can cause a puncture wound (and a punch in the nose).

FIRST AID GOALS. The priorities in wound care are: first, to control bleeding; and second, to prevent infection.

TREATMENT OF BLEEDING. The technique for stopping bleeding was covered in step three of the seven steps. Those basic methods of direct pressure, elevation, and pressure points will stop the bleeding from virtually all wounds. Placing a pressure dressing on the wound will replace direct *manual* pressure, from your hand, with *mechanical* pressure from the bandage.

Make a pressure dressing by applying several bulky sterile dressings directly over the wound, then applying a bandage snugly in place. It should be snug enough to provide pressure directly on the wound, but not so tight as to create a tourniquet by mistake. Check below the wound site after the pressure dressing is in place, to be certain that you have not stopped the circulation to the areas beyond the dressing.

Once the bleeding is under control, IMMOBILIZE the wounded part, using a splint if necessary. Further movement of the wounded area can start the bleeding again.

EMBEDDED OBJECTS. Small embedded objects just below the surface of the skin should be removed, if that can be done easily. Larger embedded objects, especially if embedded in the chest or abdomen, should be stabilized in place with numerous bulky dressings around the protruding part. Removal of a deeply embedded object can cause more injury and bleeding.

TREATMENT TO PREVENT INFECTION. For minor wounds where bleeding is not a severe problem or, for the most part, has been controlled, the wound should be cleansed and dressed under as sterile conditions as possible. The general principles of preventing infection are as follows:

1. *Wash your hands* first, and the wound second.
2. *Wash in and around the wound* to remove bacteria and other foreign matter. Any dirty wound should be washed vigorously and rinsed with large amounts of water—pour at least a quart of water over it. Antibacterial soaps, such as those containing povidone iodine (Betadyne), are useful, though not absolutely necessary if you have other soap. Some previously common antiseptics, such as mercury preparations or tincture of iodine, are harmful and should not be used.
3. *Close up the wound with a butterfly bandage* if it is gaping, but only if it is clean and small. In general, unless you are quite certain that you have thoroughly cleansed the wound, do NOT attempt to close it up—small numbers of bacteria deep in the wound can make a large infection, and infection is worse than any scar. Large gaping wounds will require evacuation for hospital care for three reasons: bleeding is generally severe; they are difficult to clean adequately in the mountaineering setting; and injury to underlying tissues will require surgical repair. *Puncture wounds* should NOT be pulled together, but should be left open and covered with a sterile dressing.

    Scalp wounds can be closed without the aid of butterflies by tying strands of hair together. Use double square knots, however, since hair has a stubborn tendency to untie.

    Butterfly bandages can be purchased commercially, or improvised from adhesive tape as shown below:

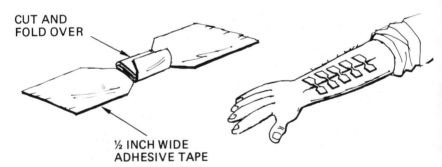

CUT AND
FOLD OVER

½ INCH WIDE
ADHESIVE TAPE

4. *Cover with a sterile dressing, and bandage.* A *bandage* holds a *dressing* in place—a bandage does not need to be sterile, but a dressing should be sterile. Gauze pad dressings in various sizes are readily available commercially. Nonadherent dressings (such as Telfa or Easy-Release pads) are particularly useful for abrasions and burns. Bandage material can be improvised (as from torn strips of clothing) or commercial (such as Kerlix or Kling). Retail *roller gauze* is cheap, but difficult to use. Two-ply *elastic gauze* (also called *self-adhering roller*

bandage) is not as cheap, but is much easier to use.

When using tape, if the skin is cold or wet and the adhesive quality of the tape is dubious, apply *tincture of benzoin* to the area around the wound. Do NOT apply tincture of benzoin to the wound itself—it is used only as an adhesive to ensure that the tape will hold. Allow the benzoin to dry before applying the tape.

5. *Change the dressing every day*, replacing it with a new dry, sterile dressing. Look for signs of infection: foul smelling pus; redness around the wound, especially if extending up the limb; swelling; fever; or considerable pain, continuing longer than two to three days. Moist heat applied over the infected wound may prove beneficial, but any significant infection is cause for evacuation as soon as possible.

6. Having an up-to-date series of shots for immunization against *tetanus* is not strictly speaking a part of first aid, but it is a key part of the *prevention* of complications.

BASIC TECHNIQUE FOR PREVENTING INFECTION

1. Wash your hands.

2. Wash in and around the wound.

3. Cover with a sterile dressing and bandage.

4. Change the dressing every day.

Head Injury

Head injuries in the mountains are caused by objects falling on the head (rockfall, icefall, and so on) or by falls in which the head strikes a hard object. All injuries to the head are potentially life threatening. Their seriousness depends on the degree of damage to the brain rather than on the visible physical damage. Scalp wounds tend to bleed profusely, so that it is easy to become alarmed over a relatively minor injury. On the other hand, serious brain injuries can be present without obvious signs or symptoms. Assessment of severity is a challenge for the first aider.

There are two basic types of head injury: *skull fracture* and *brain injury*. They are often seen together, but it is possible to have a skull fracture without brain injury or brain injury without skull fracture. A *skull fracture* is a crack or break in the bones surrounding the brain, caused by a direct blow to the head. Although a skull fracture itself is not an immediately life-threatening injury, the possibility of brain injury should be assumed whenever there has been a blow powerful enough to crack the skull.

A *brain injury* can vary in severity from a fairly minor concussion to major bleeding within the skull. A *concussion* involves temporary loss of function of some or all parts of the brain, with results ranging from mild confusion to complete loss of consciousness, followed by complete recovery. *Bleeding within the skull* is the cause of significant brain injury because the accumulating blood puts pressure on the brain. The skull is like a closed box, and an expanding blood clot will compress and injure the delicate brain tissue.

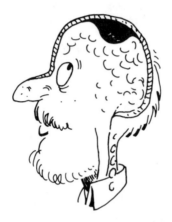

Perhaps the most important way to emphasize the significance of head injuries is to point out that BRAIN INJURIES ARE PROBABLY THE MOST COMMON CAUSE OF DEATH IN MOUNTAINEERING ACCIDENTS.

FIRST AID GOALS. The priorities of first aid for head injuries are to: prevent further injury; assess the seriousness of the injury; watch closely for changes; and evacuate as necessary.

PREVENT FURTHER INJURY. With the head-injured victim, as with any victim, the first priorities are the ABC's—airway, breathing, and circulation.

A. *Open the Airway.* Assuring an adequate airway in an unconscious victim of head injury is more difficult than usual because IT MUST BE ASSUMED THAT EVERY UNCONSCIOUS INJURED VICTIM HAS A SPINAL INJURY until proved otherwise. Approximately fifteen percent of all severe head injuries are associated with a broken neck. The number one priority is the *airway* (you may recover if nothing is done about your spine injury, but you won't recover if no one opens your airway). The *jaw thrust* (or the triple airway) techniques may be life saving.

B. *Check for Breathing.* Assure adequate breathing.

C. *Check for Circulation.* A weak pulse may indicate blood loss. A thorough head-to-toe examination is particularly important, as blood loss severe enough to cause shock usually does not result from bleeding from a head injury. Bleeding from a scalp wound can generally be controlled by direct pressure, although care should be used to avoid excess direct pressure on a head wound that is located over a skull fracture. These wounds should simply be covered with a bulky dressing, to avoid pressing fragments of bone into the brain tissue.

ASSESS SERIOUSNESS. There are six signs that distinguish a major head injury from a minor head injury:

- *Changes in consciousness* are the most obvious signs of a severe head injury. Prolonged unconsciousness, five minutes or more, is a sign of brain injury. The length of unconsciousness is roughly proportional to the seriousness of the injury. The victim who is initially knocked unconscious, wakes up, and then gradually becomes drowsy and loses consciousness again has a severe brain injury as well. This can occur when there is continued bleeding or swelling within the skull.

    It is reasonable to assume that a head injury is minor if the victim has not been knocked out, but only confused or disoriented for a very short period of time, and is now alert and oriented (knows where he or she is, the time of day, what is happening, and so on).
- Any *indentation in the skull* is a sign of a major head injury.
- *Blood or clear fluid* draining from the ears or nose is a sign of major head injury. Blood from the nose alone can result from a simple blow to the nose, so look further.
- *The appearance and function of the eyes* may be a sign of major head injury. Pupils of unequal size (see figure below) or pupils that respond unequally to light are signs of brain injury. Response to light is tested by shading the eye with the hand, then suddenly removing the hand to expose the eye to sunlight or to a flashlight. Both pupils should respond by becoming smaller equally.

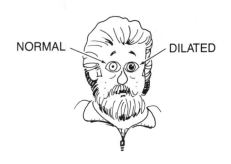

NORMAL   DILATED

Test the *function* of the eyes (sight) by asking the victim if he or she can count how many fingers you are holding up and by seeing if the victim can follow your fingers with his or her eyes as you move them upward, downward, right, and left. Difficulties with seeing may be signs of brain injury.

• *Bruises behind the ears or under the eyes* may be signs of major head injury.

• A *very slow pulse,* below forty beats per minute, is a sign of a major head injury. This is unlike shock, where a rapid pulse is a sign of seriousness.

BASIC SIGNS OF SERIOUS HEAD INJURY

- Changes in consciousness
- Indentation in the skull
- Blood or clear fluid draining from the ears or nose
- Eye pupils that respond unequally
- Bruises behind the ears or under the eyes
- Very slow pulse

WATCH CLOSELY FOR CHANGES. In the mountaineering setting, a head-injured victim may want to resume climbing after regaining consciousness. Although the victim may feel as though it is a minor injury, it is a safe rule of thumb that anyone who has been knocked out should be observed closely for the next twenty-four hours at least, and certainly not allowed to wander off alone (either up the mountain or down the trail). Keep a written record of the signs and symptoms you observe—it will be difficult to remember exact details hours later. Repeat your observations periodically (including the head-to-toe exam), as signs can change—bruises, for example, may show up only gradually. Your notes may show any progressing trends of improvement or deterioration, and may help a surgeon decide to operate within minutes of the victim's arrival at a hospital.

EVACUATE AS NECESSARY. If the victim has any of the above signs of serious head injury, then evacuation will be necessary. Use the following guidelines to help you decide whether to allow the victim to walk out:

You can allow the victim to walk out with assistance (self-evacuation) if:

• The injuries appear minor, such as very brief unconsciousness or a small scalp wound, and there are no signs of other associated injuries such as spine injury; AND

- The victim is able to walk. You can test for balance, coordination, and vision during a "trial" walk. Ask the victim to stand with eyes closed: swaying or falling may indicate injury to the brain; AND
- The terrain is safe. If portions of the trail require independent judgment and action (a rock traverse, for example, or steep, hard snow), where it is not possible for another party member to stay close, do not attempt walking out.

The tremendous difficulties involved in evacuating an unconscious victim from the backcountry are more than adequate justification for heading toward the trailhead while the victim is able to walk. When evacuating by walking, watch the victim very closely, particularly during the next six hours, for signs of drowsiness, increased headache, nausea or vomiting, which may indicate a deteriorating condition. You should EVACUATE AS SOON AS POSSIBLE when the signs and symptoms indicate a major head injury. The information you send out on the first aid report form should be sufficiently detailed to allow the professional rescuers who will be responding to decide how quickly they need to respond. If you are extremely close to the trailhead and you have a large, strong party, you may decide to attempt to carry the victim out. If you attempt to carry the victim out, the unconscious head injury victim is assumed to have a spine injury until proved otherwise, and thus the spine must be protected from any movement.

PREVENTION OF HEAD INJURIES. Severe head injuries can be virtually eliminated by use of a hard protective helmet. Helmets that are made specifically for climbers are best, because they have been designed with mountaineering accidents in mind. Bicycle helmets, for example, do not protect adequately against blows to the side of the head.

Eye Injury

Objects in the eye

Getting "something in the eye" in the mountains is common, since winds and people above you are also common. In most instances, natural watering from tears is sufficient to dislodge and wash away any object. Occasionally objects become lodged and cannot easily be removed. More rarely an object becomes embedded in the eye.

FIRST AID GOALS. The first aid goals are to remove lodged objects when possible, and to stabilize embedded objects in place.

REMOVAL. Rinsing with water may remove a foreign body lodged in the eye. With the victim horizontal, rinse from the nose side toward the ear (you want to avoid washing the object out of one eye into the other). The fluid should be poured into the inner corner of the eye and allowed to run over the eyeball while the lid is gently lifted by the lashes. The eye should not be rubbed. If rinsing fails, and the object can be seen, the first aider may try to lift it out gently with a corner of a sterile gauze pad, with the victim looking away. If the object is embedded, leave it in place and bandage the eye.

STABILIZE EMBEDDED OBJECTS. If an object is embedded in or protruding from the eye, the situation clearly is much more serious. The object needs to be stabilized in place because movement could cause fluid from the inside of the eye to be lost, and once lost it can never be replaced. Follow these steps:

1. Leave the object in place. Do not attempt to wash the eye.
2. Using a cravat or clothing, improvise a "doughnut" or "bagel" to encircle the protruding object.

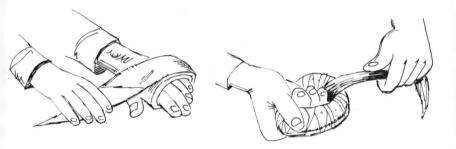

3. Place a bandage over both eyes, being careful not to disturb the protruding object. It is necessary to cover both eyes because they move together, and eye movement in the uninjured eye will cause pain and more harm to the injured eye.

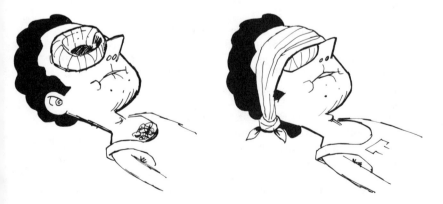

4. Evacuate the victim by stretcher when both eyes are covered. Under extreme conditions, such as increasing avalanche risk, it may be necessary to walk out of a hazardous area. In this case, after the impaled object is stabilized, the uninjured eye can be covered with a shield of cardboard or similar opaque material with a small hole in the center. This type of shield permits the patient to see only straight ahead and minimizes eye movements, thereby tending to splint the injured eye.

Snowblindness

Snowblindness is not "blindness" at all, but rather sunburn of the surface of the eye. The atmosphere, which screens out most of the harmful ultraviolet rays, is thinner at higher altitudes, and thus mountaineers are at greater risk of sunburn. The surface of the eye is probably more sensitive to ultraviolet radiation than the skin, and travel on snow (which reflects much of the UV rays) can cause injury to the eyes if they are not properly protected. This injury is identical to what is commonly called "arc welder's burn." Just as in sunburn, the injury does not become obvious until several hours after the exposure.

FIRST AID GOALS. The first aid priorities for snowblindness are: first, to recognize that the problem is snowblindness and not something else; second, to prevent further injury; and third, to relieve pain.

RECOGNITION. Snowblindness is recognized more by the symptoms reported by the victim than by the objective physical signs. All that is visible to the observer are eyes that are bloodshot and tearing. The victim may report having traveled on a snowfield earlier in the day, and will initially complain of eyes that feel simply irritated or dry. Some victims mistakenly believe that there is merely an object in the eye. Severe symptoms are: feeling as if the eyes are "full of sand" and pain when moving or blinking the eyes.

PREVENT FURTHER INJURY. As soon as the problem is recognized, action must be taken to prevent further injury by protecting the eyes from further exposure to the sun. Dark goggles or sunglasses with side shields are useful. Using both together is best for someone with initial symptoms of snowblindness. The protection of a single pair of sunglasses can be improved by placing tape over the lenses, leaving a horizontal slit to see through. Side shields can also be improvised, as can a "Lone Ranger" style mask with narrow slits, made from cardboard or similar material. Covering the eyes entirely may be necessary for someone with severe symptoms, although that will necessitate leading the now actually "blind" person by the hand, or possibly mean evacuation by stretcher.

PAIN RELIEF. Pain can be relieved by cool wet compresses. Aspirin can be helpful as well. Anesthetic ointments are inadvisable, as they can cause further injury if the victim rubs the eyes. As with any sunburn, rubbing is not a good idea. Patching the eyes firmly, so that they cannot open under the patches, provides good relief of pain.

PREVENTION. Having and wearing sunglasses that screen out ninety percent or more of the UV light and have side shields is the best prevention of snowblindness. It is also a good idea to carry an emergency pair of collapsible dark goggles.

Neck and Back Injuries: Damage to the Spine

The *spinal column* is a column of bones extending from the skull to the pelvis. The *spinal cord* is encased within the column, and nerves branch off of the cord to go to the arms, the trunk, and the legs. These nerves and the cord carry sensory messages up to the brain and motor (movement) messages down from the brain. Damage to the spinal cord interrupts those messages, resulting in the inability to sense or move. A *spinal fracture* is a break or crack in the bones of the spinal column. These fractures can occur with or without injury to the spinal cord.

Spinal injuries can result from a direct blow to the spine, or from a blow to the head or fall on the buttocks (which transmits the force indirectly to the spine). Falls and falling rock are the most common causes in the mountains.

The most vulnerable areas of the spinal column are the neck and lower back; the upper back is somewhat strengthened by its connection to the rib cage. A spinal fracture in the neck or back causes instability, and therefore less protection for the cord. Mishandling of a spinal injury can convert a spinal column fracture that has not resulted in spinal cord damage into one that has. The sharp, jagged broken bone edges can easily cut into the cord. Mishandling can also convert a partially cut cord into a totally cut cord. The nerve cells in the spinal cord are almost entirely incapable of healing; therefore, spinal damage is permanent.

All things considered, the case of spinal injury is probably the best example of why we repeatedly say in first aid: "it is better to overtreat than to undertreat." If there is any doubt about whether a spinal injury exists, it is always best to assume it does and handle accordingly. The person who is immobilized unnecessarily suffers little harm, but the person who has a minor spinal injury converted into a major injury through mishandling may suffer permanent paralysis.

FIRST AID GOALS. The first aid goals for spinal injury are to: assess the seriousness of the injury; prevent further injury; and monitor and evacuate.

ASSESS SERIOUSNESS. The victim of a neck or back injury may have sustained a fracture of the spinal column without serious injury (yet) to the spinal cord. For that reason, *any sign or symptom which is suggestive of spinal injury should be taken to mean that immobilization of the spine is necessary.* Similarly, *when the mechanism of injury* (fall, blow to the head, etc.) *suggests damage to the spine,* IMMOBILIZE THE VICTIM. With the victim immobilized, repeat your observations every twenty minutes or so: the signs and symptoms may not have been obvious the first time you checked, and some victims may not develop them until later. It is safe to

Signs and Symptoms of Spinal Injury

	NECK	BACK
SYMPTOMS		
pain	in the neck	in the back
numbness, tingling	fingers	toes
loss of sensation	arms	legs
SIGNS		
tenderness	neck	back
deformity	neck	back
loss of movement	fingers	toes

assume that no spinal injury is present only when NONE of the symptoms or signs are present.

The location of the injury determines the signs and symptoms that can be found. The victim may report the following symptoms: pain at the site (neck or back), numbness or tingling of the fingers or toes, or a loss of sensation. Signs that may be found include: tenderness or deformity at the site (neck or back), or a loss of the ability to move the arms or legs. Carefully record the place on the body where the loss of sensation or ability to move occurs.

The specific test for sensation and movement of the upper body involves three steps: 1) touch the skin and ask if the victim feels it; 2) tell the victim to wiggle his or her fingers; and then 3) tell the victim to squeeze your hand. For the lower body, the approach is similar: 1) touch the skin and ask if the victim feels it; 2) tell the victim to wiggle his or her toes; and then 3) tell the victim to push down with his or her foot against your hand. When the injury is in the neck, both the arms and legs will be affected. When the injury is in the back, only the legs will be affected. If a change is found in only a single arm or a single leg, the damage is usually not to the spine, but rather to nerves outside the spinal column.

TESTING FOR SENSATION AND MOVEMENT

UPPER BODY	LOWER BODY
1. Touch hand and ask: *Can you feel this?*	Touch foot and ask: *Can you feel this?*
2. Ask: *Can you wiggle your fingers?*	Ask: *Can you wiggle your toes?*
3. Have victim squeeze your hand.	Have victim push against your hand with foot.

PREVENT FURTHER INJURY. When the symptoms or signs suggest that a spinal injury may be present, the first step is manual immobilization of the spine: hold the victim in place so that he or she does not roll or slide or move in any way. As with any victim, the ABC's of airway, breathing, and circulation take priority. Whenever a neck injury is suspected, the jaw thrust should be used to open the airway.

With a possible broken neck, stabilize the head in the position found unless you are unable to keep the airway open; if so, straighten by applying tension (gentle pulling) in the direction of the long axis of the body. The hands are positioned with fingers placed supporting the back of the head and the thumbs over the jaw. The palms typically cover the ears, with the hands in this position, as is shown in figure below. A mountaineering helmet may be left in place while stabilizing the neck. If a helmet must be removed (e.g. to care for a wound), it should be done by two people: one to hold the head and neck stable while the other removes the helmet.

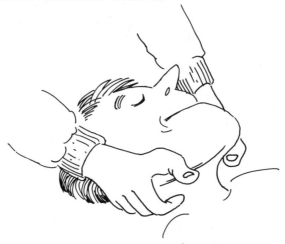

STABILIZING THE NECK

The next priority is to protect the victim from heat loss by placing insulation underneath him or her. Victims of spinal injury are particularly sensitive to changes in temperature. The insulation should be slid under the victim, or the victim rolled as a unit (the "logroll" is covered in detail in Chapter 4).

When it is no longer necessary to move the victim, replace the manual immobilization with a method that does not require you to hold the person constantly. The best method for a suspected neck fracture in the mountaineering setting involves improvising "sandbags" using stuff sacks filled with dirt (or clothing) or with tightly rolled bulky clothing around the head, neck and shoulders. This "sandbag" arrangement can then be anchored in place by positioning stones or rocks against it, or with a tie.

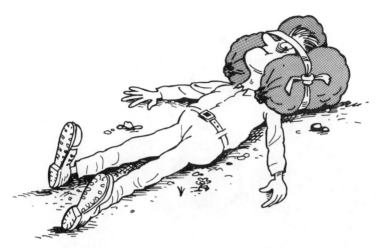

STABILIZATION WITH "SANDBAGS"

MONITOR AND EVACUATE. Watch the victim for changes. Many victims will have further loss in sensation or ability to move over time. Evacuation of a victim of a spinal injury must be by rigid stretcher. It is not possible to improvise a rigid stretcher with ropes or other typical mountaineering gear, so you will have to wait for an organized rescue party.

Chest Injuries

Puncture Wounds of the Chest

Chest injuries cause one out of four deaths from trauma in the United States, and a chest injury in the mountains is thus a particular cause for concern. Any penetrating injury to the chest can cause a puncture wound. A penetrating injury to the chest can result from a fall onto a sharp object, such as a sharp rock, or an ice axe in an improperly performed ice axe arrest.

A puncture wound can cause a collapsed lung and death from a lack of oxygen. In normal respiration the chest expands and air is drawn in the mouth and nose. When the chest relaxes, the air is pushed out. A hole in the chest from a puncture wound can create another route for the air to go in and out, causing a "sucking sound." When part or all of a lung collapses, the victim experiences difficulty breathing and thus gets less oxygen.

FIRST AID GOALS. The goals of first aid for a puncture wound to the chest are to: assess the seriousness of the injury; prevent further injury; help increase the ease of breathing; and watch closely for changes.

ASSESS SERIOUSNESS. A serious puncture wound to the chest can kill someone just about as quickly as a severed artery, which means that it is

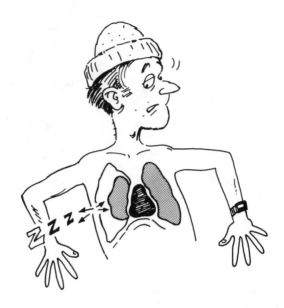

important to assess the seriousness of the wound as soon as possible. When a chest injury is suspected, it will be necessary to bare the chest in order to look and listen. If you need to turn the victim over to see and treat the wound, then stabilize embedded objects (and/or the victim's neck) as the victim is rolled over. When there is a sucking wound, the sucking sound can be heard on both inhalation and exhalation.

PREVENT FURTHER INJURY. In order to keep the victim's condition from worsening, follow these steps.

1. Seal the hole as quickly as possible, with your bare hand if necessary.
2. Cover the wound with a sterile dressing, one that is several times larger than the hole itself (in order to avoid it being sucked into the hole).
3. Cover the dressing with an *occlusive dressing* of some kind. An occlusive dressing is one that blocks the flow of air, and so is made from such material as plastic or foil. Put it in place to make the seal at the end of exhalation.
4. Tape the dressing in place with tape on all four sides.
5. Stabilize any embedded object, if necessary.

HELP INCREASE THE EASE OF BREATHING. Lay the victim

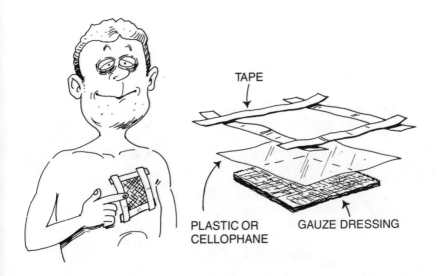

TAPE

PLASTIC OR CELLOPHANE   GAUZE DRESSING

on the injured side, as this allows the uninjured lung to work more effectively.

WATCH CLOSELY FOR CHANGES. Observe the victim at regular intervals, and especially ask if the person seems to be having increased difficulty breathing. If so, the occlusive dressing may have to be checked to make sure air is not being trapped inside the chest and exerting pressure on the lungs and heart. IF TRAPPED AIR ESCAPES AND THE VICTIM FEELS IMMEDIATE RELIEF WHEN THE SEAL IS LIFTED BRIEFLY, THEN THE SEAL MAY NEED TO BE VENTED AT INTERVALS. Use the victim's condition as your guide.

FIRST AID METHOD FOR PUNCTURE WOUND OF THE CHEST

1. Seal the wound.
2. Cover with a sterile dressing.
3. Cover the dressing with an occlusive dressing.
4. Tape in place.
5. Watch closely for changes.

Rib Fractures

A fracture is a break or crack in a bone. The major symptom of rib fracture is pain, localized over the injured area, which is worse with deep breathing. Signs are deformity and bruising, but these may be subtle or absent.

Rib fractures vary in severity from a simple single broken rib to multiple ribs broken in several places. Most rib fractures are caused by falls.

FIRST AID GOALS. The goals of first aid for rib fractures are to: assess the seriousness of the injury; help increase the ease of breathing; and watch closely for changes.

ASSESS SERIOUSNESS. Look for the number of ribs involved, and get down to bare skin to do so. If you find an open wound, put a dressing on it as indicated. Observe how deeply (or shallowly) the victim is breathing.

HELP INCREASE THE EASE OF BREATHING. When there are one or two broken ribs, an improvised pillow, such as a rolled sweater, can be placed over the injured area for comfort. The victim can hold it in place, if desired.

When there are three or more ribs fractured, act as follows:

1. Place thick padding, such as some tightly rolled clothing, over the injured area.
2. Tape the pad in place or bind it to the chest with three or four cravats. Tighten the cravats as the victim exhales. Do not tie so tightly as to restrict ability to breathe.
3. Position the victim to help ease breathing: sitting is likely to be the most comfortable position. Some victims may not be able to sit, such as those in shock. In that case, place the victim with the injured side down.

WATCH CLOSELY FOR CHANGES. Stabilizing broken ribs, as outlined above, should reduce the pain and make breathing easier. The victim should also be encouraged to breathe as deeply as possible to avoid the possibility of developing a pneumonia.

PREVENTION OF CHEST INJURIES. Both types of chest injury can be related to the use (or misuse) of equipment: ice axes and ropes. Proper use of the ice axe and seat harness can be learned during adequate training in ice axe arrest and roped travel. A once common cause of rib fracture, falling while roped with a bowline so that the coil slips up over the ribs, is now less frequent, with the increased use of seat harnesses. Leather or rubber guards over the sharp pick, adze, and spike of an ice axe can prevent injury. Individual guards can be removed one at a time as conditions warrant (the adze cover, for example, rarely needs to be removed except when chopping steps in hard snow or ice).

Abdominal Injuries

Open wounds to the abdomen can be obvious, particularly when there are protruding intestines. Closed wounds to the abdomen may be more difficult to detect. In the mountains, open wounds to the abdomen can be caused by an ice axe or a ski pole. Wound care is the same as in any other open wound, with one exception: an occlusive dressing should be placed over the sterile dressing to prevent drying out of the abdominal contents. The victim may be more comfortable lying with the knees bent.

A closed injury to the abdomen is less obvious, and thus may be more dangerous, since it can delay recognition of a life-threatening injury. You should suspect injury to the internal organs of the abdomen when the mechanism of injury, such as the distance fallen, suggests that it is possible. The signs of internal injury may be subtle, and close attention should be paid to the signs and symptoms of shock. Although other signs may be seen, such as bruising, abdominal rigidity or tenderness, the development of shock may be the first indication of serious injury. First aid in the mountains is limited to close observation of the victim and evacuation as soon as possible. As with head injury, a careful written record of the signs and symptoms you observe may be very useful to the surgeon in the hospital.

Extremity Injuries

Fractures, Dislocations, and Sprains

Bones come together at joints, which in turn are held together by ligaments. A break or crack in a bone is called a *fracture*. When a bone end is displaced from a joint, it is called a *dislocation*. When a joint is bent beyond its limits and a ligament is torn, it is called a *sprain*. A *strain,* on the other hand, is simply an overstretched muscle.

Like wounds, fractures are classified as either closed or open, depending on whether the skin is broken. An open fracture can result from either a direct blow or from an indirect force, such as a twisting injury, causing the broken bone end to push through the skin.

Fractures can be recognized by symptoms and signs. The victim will report pain and a loss of the ability to use the extremity, and possibly may report having heard or felt a snap or crack. The examiner will find deformity (compare to the uninjured side), tenderness around the full circumference of the limb, swelling, instability, bruising (later), and possibly may hear a grating sound. Because blood vessels and nerves travel alongside the bone, jagged bone ends can cause serious damage. First aid for fractures is splinting.

Dislocations occur at joints, most commonly at the shoulder or hip. The victim will report pain and a loss of the ability to use the joint. The examiner will find deformity, tenderness, and occasionally swelling. The joint may seem "locked" in position. Similar to fractures, the potential exists for the displaced bone end to cut off circulation or impinge on nerves. First aid for dislocations is splinting.

Sprains also occur at joints, most commonly at the ankle or knee. The victim will report pain, aggravated by motion. The examiner will find localized tenderness and swelling. First aid for sprains is rest, ice, compression, and elevation (R.I.C.E.).

It can be difficult, especially in the mountaineering setting, to tell precisely whether an injury is a fracture, a dislocation, or a sprain. It is even difficult at times for doctors in a hospital to tell, which is why they have X-ray machines. In fact, dislocations often have associated fractures. So, if you have any doubt, ALWAYS TREAT AN EXTREMITY INJURY AS IF A FRACTURE WERE PRESENT. (Unless, of course, you can see whether a fracture is present because you have X-ray vision, like Superman....)

FIRST AID GOALS. The first aid goals for extremity injuries are to assess the seriousness of the injury; to prevent further injury by reducing movement; and to control pain.

ASSESS SERIOUSNESS. The total victim comes first, and the ABC's of airway, breathing, and circulation take priority. It is easy to become so involved with a gruesome extremity injury that the needs of the total patient are neglected. A fracture can wait. The airway cannot.

Assess the victim for the signs and symptoms of shock. A fracture of the pelvis or femur (upper leg) often results in shock.

Assessment of the seriousness of the extremity injury requires baring the skin for a good look at it. You may have to remove several layers, or cut some clothes. You may miss an open fracture if you do not get down to bare skin.

A serious complication of an extremity injury can result from the fact that blood vessels and nerves travel alongside the bone, and may be injured by jagged bone ends. Thus *examination of the victim must include a check for a pulse beyond the site of the injury.* When the injury has affected the blood flow, evacuation must be as soon as possible.

PREVENT FURTHER INJURY. The basic principle for preventing further injury is immobilization. This can range from the temporary immobilization for a suspected sprained joint (R.I.C.E.) to rigid immobilization for a suspected fracture.

Naturally, this may interfere with your alpine travel plans. Using R.I.C.E. on a suspected sprain of the ankle or knee may allow the victim to walk out under his or her own steam (self-evacuation), but the potential exists for making the injury worse. What is suspected of being a sprain may actually be a fracture. In general, let pain be your guide. If the injury is too painful to walk on, then don't walk on it.

You may need to wait one to one-and-a-half hours before making the decision about walking out, but there is no advantage to getting a short distance down the trail to where you don't want to be and then not being able to go any farther.

The basic rule of immobilization of an extremity injury is to immobilize both adjacent joints. Thus, if the forearm is injured, immobilize the wrist and the elbow (and the forearm between). If the knee is injured, immobilize the ankle and the hip.

Splinting

GENERAL PRINCIPLES OF SPLINTING. Having an organized approach to splinting is essential (as with most procedures in first aid). DON'T JUST DO SOMETHING, STAND THERE (and figure out what you are going to do).

1. *Determine the extent of the injury* by looking and feeling, both at the injury site and below. Check for a pulse, and assess sensation and movement below the injury (fingers or toes).
2. If there is an open fracture, *stop the bleeding* with direct pressure. Put a dressing on all open wounds before applying a splint.
3. If there are exposed bone ends which are covered with dirt and debris, the *dirt should be rinsed off* with large amounts of water. To reduce the likelihood of infection, it is best to use water that has been previously boiled. It takes some time to boil water and then wait for it to cool enough to use. If evacuation is expected to be prolonged, taking the time may be quite worthwhile, as the objective is to reduce the probability of an infected wound.
4. IF the extremity is *severely bent out of its normal shape* (angulated) and IF the injury is *not at a joint,* THEN *pull on the limb to straighten it.* When the limb is severely angulated, it may be difficult to apply a splint. In addition, a severely angulated injury can cut off circulation. The advice "splint them where they lie" means that the person is not to be moved. The limb occasionally must be moved to restore normal position, especially when there is a badly distorted break. A steady, firm, but gentle pull in the direction of the long axis of the extremity is applied while the trunk is supported by another person.

    IF the injury is at a joint (for example, the elbow or the knee) AND IF there is no pulse below (and the hand or foot is cold and discolored), THEN *pull gently to straighten* it until a pulse returns. The limb should *not* be straightened when there is a suspected dislocation and the circulation below the joint is good.
5. *Prepare a splint* that is of appropriate material, the right size, and well padded. Splints, which can be either improvised or commercial, can also be either rigid or soft. Rigid splints can be improvised from a pack-frame stay, an ice axe, tent poles, a spare ski tip, or tightly rolled closed cell foam. A makeshift sling can be improvised by using safety pins to pin a sleeve to

BASIC PRINCIPLES OF SPLINTING

1. Determine the extent of the injury.
2. Stop bleeding, where necessary.
3. Rinse dirt off exposed bone ends, cover with sterile dressing.
4. Straighten badly angulated limbs by gentle pulling.
5. Prepare a splint, size it, and pad it.
6. Tie the splint on.
7. Observe below the site for circulation and sensation.
8. Elevate the injured extremity.
9. Apply cold compresses to the injury site.

the front of the jacket. You could even use this first aid book as a rigid splint (although once you have tied it on the victim you can't look anything up). Tree branches are overrated as sources for splints, as they are difficult to remove from trees if they are still attached, are generally brittle and easily broken if they are not still attached to the tree, and are nonexistent above timberline. Many mountaineers carry a light, moldable "ladder splint," which avoids tying up some other object (such as your ice axe) that may have another important use. When there is absolutely nothing available for improvising a splint, or when there may not be enough time to construct a splint, as in an emergency rescue situation, you can always tie an injured extremity to an uninjured part of the body. Tie a broken leg to a good leg, or bind an arm to the chest.

A splint of the right size must be long enough to immobilize the joint above and the joint below the injury. Measure the uninjured extremity to estimate the proper size. The final step in preparing the splint is making sure that it is well padded. Be certain to fill hollows, such as inside the palm of the hand or at the ankle. A splint must evenly support an injured extremity throughout its entire length, exerting equal pressure on both protrusions and hollows, so that the limb will not move inside the splint.

6. *Tie the splint on* gently but firmly: too loose and the splint will fall off; too tight and you will have accidentally created a tourniquet. The ties should be on either side of the injury, as well as next to the adjacent joints. Tie the knots in an accessible place.

7. *Observe areas below the injury site* for circulation and sensation, and repeat this observation at least every half hour. If the victim

complains of numbness or tingling in the fingers or toes (or is unable to straighten them), then check the tightness of the ties immediately. Swelling may make your "just right" ties become too tight, and they may have to be loosened. Obviously, fingertips and toes need to be accessible for these observations.

8. When possible, *elevate the injured extremity*. Elevation can slow the development of swelling.

9. If the victim is warm, cold compresses can be applied to the injury site, which will reduce pain and also delay swelling.

SPECIFIC PROCEDURES FOR IMMOBILIZATION. These specific instructions for splinting use the principles explained in Steps 5 and 6 above.

Upper Extremities: the *sling and swathe*. The sling supports the arm in place, and is useful for fractures of both the collarbone and the arm, but does not by itself immobilize either the elbow joint or the shoulder joint. The swathe binds the arm in place to the body.

a. When possible, place a rigid splint over the injury, as with a suspected forearm fracture or upper arm fracture.

b. Position the arm across the chest, with the wrist slightly higher than the elbow.

c. Position the triangular bandage with the long side by the hand and the opposite point at the elbow. The fingertips should be just barely visible, extending beyond the edge of the sling, to allow for checking circulation.

d. Tie a knot at the side of the neck, and place a pad underneath.

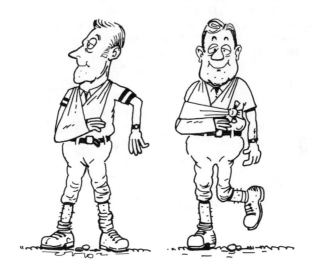

e. Pin or tie the elbow end, to form a pocket for the elbow.
f. Place the swathe across the chest, horizontally. It should be fairly wide where it goes over the injured arm.

Lower Extremities: the "pillow" splint for an injured ankle. This is a soft splint, and allows the victim to protect the injured area with a maximum of comfort.

a. Wrap a bulky jacket or vest around the foot and ankle.
b. Tie it in place with at least three ties. (Safety pins make an acceptable substitute if cravats are unavailable.)

Lower Extremities: rigid splint for a lower leg injury.

a. Choose, size, and pad the splint, as described above. If an ice axe is used, the spike end should be pointing toward the waist and the pick up (adze down). This position allows for the ankle to be secured to the ice-axe head.
b. Deciding whether to leave the boot on or remove it can be a hard choice. The foot may need protection from the possibility of frostbite if you are in an exposed place or on snow, but it is critical to have access to the toes to check circulation periodically. Having a boot on the foot is really only absolutely necessary when the victim intends to walk on it, and a down bootie and/or several pairs of socks can be used for protection from the elements. It is possible to cut an inspection hole in the tip of the socks, and cover the toes with another sock. Then only the one sock over the toes needs to be removed to check circulation, without disturbing the entire splint.
c. Place the padded splint next to the injured leg. With a knee injury, you may decide to place the splint under the leg.
d. Tie in place with at least four ties.

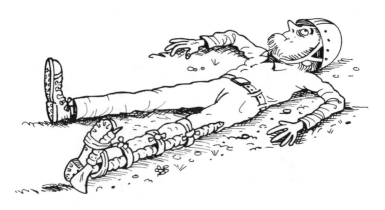

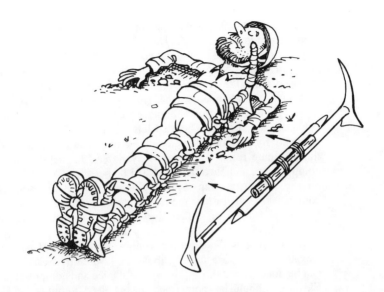

Lower Extremities: rigid splint for an upper leg injury. A suspected fracture of the upper leg is a challenge to splint well. A sturdy splint can be made from two ice axes tied together with a third support, as shown in the diagram below. The third piece, which can be a tent pole, ski pole, or whatever, adds to the stability considerably.

    a. Choose, size, and pad the splint. The splint should extend from the armpit to below the ankle.

    b. The same considerations regarding removing the boot apply as discussed above.

    c. Put the splint in place. You may decide to add another splint on the inside of the leg for further support.

    d. Pad between the legs.

    e. Tie in place with a minimum of seven ties, five on the leg. The ties on the body are meant to immobilize the hip joint, and to discourage the victim from trying to sit up.

    f. When possible, evacuate by rigid stretcher. The ice axe splint alone does not completely immobilize the hip.

Rest, Ice, Compression, and Elevation (R.I.C.E.)

First aid for sprains and strains consists of a sequence of four steps, designed to reduce the damage and the swelling.

Rest. After an injury has occurred, stop. Continuing to use an injured arm or leg can result in extending the amount of damage done. Walking on a badly twisted knee or ankle can result in further damage and lead to a much prolonged recovery time. After an injury, stop and give the joint a chance to rest.

Ice. A bag of crushed ice, or a stuff sack filled with snow, should be wrapped around the injured area. The application of cold will reduce the development of swelling and speed recovery. To protect the part from frostbite, place a layer of cloth between the cold pack and the skin. The ice is left in place for thirty minutes, removed for ten minutes, and then reapplied for a second thirty-minute time. (If no ice is available, the steps of rest, compression, and elevation will still be beneficial.)

Compression. An elastic wrap can be applied over the ice bag, and the compression will further reduce the development of swelling. Check below the level of the injury for pulses to ensure that the elastic wrap has not been too tightly applied.

Elevation. Swelling will be further limited if the injured part is elevated to a position slightly above the level of the heart. This can be done during the application of the ice and compression. Elevation should be maintained during the ten-minute break between ice applications.

After the two thirty-minute ice applications, the injury can be reevaluated for seriousness. If the signs and symptoms indicate that the injury is limited to a sprain or strain, the injured person may try to use the part. When using the injured part, every effort should be made to use as natural motions as possible. Walking with a limp can place much greater stress on the joint. Using a natural motion puts the least amount of strain on the injured area. The injured person should carry as little weight as possible. If severe pain remains or if pain increases, the part should again receive the R.I.C.E. treatment and further use should be delayed until another day.

Burns

Burns can be classified according to severity or degree. A *first-degree burn* involves reddening of the skin, mild pain, and slight swelling. The average sunburn is a typical first-degree burn. A *second-degree burn* involves blistering of the skin, mild to moderate pain, and moderate swelling (over a period of days). A scald from boiling hot water is a typical second-degree burn. A *third-degree burn* involves damage to the skin and underlying tissues; it may appear white or charred, and causes moderate to severe pain. A lightning injury or prolonged exposure to a flame can cause a third-degree burn.

The severity of a burn is also related to its location. In particular, any burn of the face or head may indicate serious injury to the breathing passages. Similarly, the extent of the burn affects its severity: a very small third-degree burn is about as bad as a much larger second-degree burn.

FIRST AID GOALS. The priorities in burn care are: first, to prevent further injury or contamination; second, to relieve pain; and third, to assess and treat other injuries.

PREVENTION OF FURTHER INJURY. First, PUT OUT THE FIRE! Pour water on the burned area or immerse it in water, unless the burn is quite old. There may still be enough heat retained in the burned tissues, or in smoldering clothing, to continue to make the damage worse. Remove all burned clothing. Small fragments of adhered cloth should *not* be removed from the burn wound.

With a minor burn, where the skin is intact. If the burn is first degree or second degree with unbroken blisters, the burned area can be immersed in cold water to relieve the pain. The part can remain immersed for thirty minutes, or until the pain subsides. Afterwards, blisters should be protected by covering with a dry sterile dressing.

With a major burn, where the skin is broken. If the burn is second degree with broken blisters or is suspected to be third degree, then the burn care is as follows:

1. Once the fire is out, carefully wash the burned area with a sterile gauze pad, soap, and previously boiled water.
2. Remove all rings or other tight jewelry from the affected area.
3. Apply a dry, sterile dressing.
4. Pain can be relieved by wrapping the burned area with an *occlusive* dressing (such as plastic wrap) to exclude air. Ice packs may also be used, over the plastic, for pain relief—but avoid overcooling the victim.
5. Elevate a burned extremity.
6. Assess the victim thoroughly. Look for signs and symptoms of shock, and treat if necessary. A particularly thorough physical examination is necessary in the case of a victim of lightning injury, because the electrical current passes through the body, causing extensive damage to tissues on its way. Look specifically for an entrance wound and an exit wound, and treat as any burn wound. Be aware that fractures are common. Similarly, head and facial burns require especially thorough physical examination and monitoring.
7. Any suspected third-degree burn or second-degree burn of over fifteen percent of the body surface area should be evacuated as soon as possible. (Fifteen percent is roughly the size of the front of the chest, or the front of both arms together.)

When evacuation is not indicated, or is not possible, then change the dressing every day, as with any other wound. Look for signs of infection (see "Treatment to Prevent Infection" in Chapter 3). Nonadherent dressings (such as Telfa or Easy-Release pads) are particularly useful.

BASIC FIRST AID FOR MAJOR BURNS

1. Once the fire is out, wash the burned area.
2. Remove rings.
3. Apply a dry, sterile dressing.
4. Wrap in an occlusive dressing.
5. Elevate a burned extremity.
6. Assess the victim thoroughly.
7. Evacuate as indicated.

There are a number of *don't's* in burn care—old practices that have been discarded as a result of medical research. *Don't* break blisters or remove tissue. *Don't* put any kind of "antiseptic" goo on a burn. In fact, don't put any kind of goo on a burn. *Don't* put snow or ice directly on the burn wound. Frostbite and hypothermia are unwanted complications.

PREVENTION. The worst burns in mountaineering occur when a tent catches fire with someone inside. Cook outside of tents whenever possible, and always position stoves so that escape is easy if an unexpected fire begins. Most tents sold today use flame retardant materials, but not all do. When purchasing your next tent, check. In addition, special care should be taken in the handling of stoves and fuels.

The most frequent burns in the mountains are *sunburns*. Travel across snowfields or glaciers can be a source of particularly severe sunburns on a sunny day. Reflected light can burn the inside of your mouth or the underside of your nose. Sunburn to the tissue covering the eye, called *snowblindness,* can be a miserable and disabling event. Even a seemingly cloudy day can cause a bad burn.

Prevention of sunburn is more effective than any first aid that can be administered. For the first outing of the season on snow, for example, an exposure of more than fifteen minutes without protection should be avoided. Later in the season, after tanning, the exposure time may be lengthened. Lightweight hats, scarves, or handkerchiefs worn about the head also provide protection from sunburn. No matter how bizarre the effect, the use of hats and scarves can be very worthwhile. Additionally, you can use protective creams or ointments. These come in two types: *opaque*, such as zinc oxide or clown white; and *sunscreen*, such as those containing the chemical PABA. Because individuals vary widely in their tolerance to sun exposure (from fair-haired, light-skinned, easily-burned to dark-haired, dark-skinned, easily-tanned), sunscreens come in different ratings. You should choose a preparation that is rated for your skin type. In addition, be careful to choose a sun-blocking agent that will not dissolve in perspiration or rub off easily.

SHOCK

Shock is a process resulting from collapse of the system of heart and blood vessels. Shock can usually be expected in any major injury associated with loss of blood or other fluids. It may be found with injuries to the spine or with severe allergic reactions. Shock results in insufficient movement of blood to provide adequate nutrients and oxygen to the tissues of the body.

The victim in shock becomes restless and anxious as the level of oxygen delivered to the brain is lowered. The pulse rate increases as the heart labors to supply a decreased amount of blood to major organs. As blood is directed to internal organs, the skin becomes pale. Waste products are not removed from the tissues. All usual functions of the body are affected.

Care given during the early stages of shock may prevent further worsening of this condition and save the victim's life. If severe shock is not treated promptly, death occurs. Any victim found with severe symptoms of shock should IMMEDIATELY be evacuated to a hospital.

Treatment for shock begins early, before a complete check for injuries has been finished. The victim's body heat must be maintained by covering the victim and providing insulation from the cold ground. In a hot environment the victim may need to be protected from excessive heat. Any victim who shows decreased awareness of the surroundings or decreased sensation to pain or touch should be examined carefully for other injuries.

Further treatment includes positioning the victim with as little movement as possible. The lower extremities may be raised twelve inches to aid in circulation of blood to the core of the body. Patients having shortness of breath may be more comfortable in a semi-upright position. Severe shock may indicate a need for movement before other injuries are treated.

Signs and Symptoms of Shock

EARLY SIGNS	EARLY SYMPTOMS
• Restlessness	• Thirstiness
• Face may be pale, dull ashen gray or yellowish brown	• Nausea
• Pulse is rapid	• Anxiety

LATER SIGNS	LATER SYMPTOMS
• Skin is cold and damp	• Lethargy and apathy
• Breathing may be shallow, rapid	
• Pulse is weak, irregular	
• Eyes become dull, pupils dilated	

65

FIRST AID FOR SHOCK

---

1. Keep the victim's airway open and clear.
2. Control all obvious bleeding.
3. Maintain the victim's body temperature.
4. Position the victim to aid in the circulation of blood to the core and to aid breathing.
5. Avoid rough or excessive handling of the victim.
6. Frequently take and record the victim's vital signs.
7. Evacuate the victim to medical care.

If the victim is to be rescued and taken to a hospital in a few hours, do not administer fluids or food. If evacuation will be delayed, a slightly salted solution may be given in sips. Bouillon dissolved in warm water is an excellent fluid, as are electrolyte replacement drinks sold for athletes.

ILLNESSES RELATED TO ENVIRONMENT: COLD, HEAT, AND ALTITUDE

Excessive heat, cold, exposure to high altitude, and overexertion in the mountain environment may lead to many painful but usually avoidable illnesses. Prevention of these illnesses is based in a knowledge of the mechanisms leading to illness, adequate care in consumption of food and water, strong physical conditioning, and a continual awareness of changes taking place within and around the mountaineer.

Effects of Excessive Cold

Hypothermia

Hypothermia is a condition in which the temperature of the body's internal core has been lowered sufficiently to cause illness. Hypothermia is dangerous in its absence of warning to the victim, and in its early effects on judgment and reasoning. The victim is quickly unable to recognize the condition. Unless a companion recognizes symptoms and begins treatment, this vicious cycle leads to apathy, collapse, and death. Hypothermia is not a condition of cold weather alone. Many hypothermia cases are reported in wet, windy weather with temperatures well above freezing. Falling in a glacial crevasse or being wetted by a cold stream can quickly bring about severe hypothermia.

It is useful to review some basic concepts of how the body can gain and lose heat. The body gains or conserves heat in four ways:

- Through the *digestion of food*. The body produces heat by digestion of food to maintain normal body temperatures.
- From the *external application of heat*. Examples of this are sun, fire, and warmth from another body.
- From *muscular activity,* either by deliberate exercise or by involuntary exercise like shivering. Shivering produces as much heat as running at a slow pace.
- Through *reduction of blood flow* near the surface of the body. Constriction of surface blood vessels reduces circulation at the skin layers and blood is kept nearer to the central core of the body. Warmth is preserved for the core organs of the body: brain, heart, and lungs.

The body loses heat in the following ways:

- *Evaporation*. Evaporation of perspiration from the skin and fluid from the lungs during breathing contributes greatly to the amount of heat lost by the body.
- *Conduction*. Sitting on the snow, touching cold equipment, and being rained upon are all examples of how heat can be lost as a result of conduction.
- *Radiation* causes the greatest amount of heat loss from uncovered surfaces of the body. The head and neck, areas where large blood vessels come close to the surface of the body, are particularly susceptible to heat loss.
- *Convection*. The body continually warms, by radiation, a thin layer of air next to the skin. If the warm air remains close to the body, an insulation effect is provided. If this layer is removed by wind or air currents, cooling takes place at a much more rapid pace.

CHANGES IN THE BODY DURING HYPOTHERMIA. If heat loss exceeds heat gain, and this situation is allowed to continue, hypothermia results. The first response to exposure to cold is constriction of the blood vessels of the skin, and later, of the deeper lying tissues. The effect is to decrease the amount of heat transported by blood to the skin, consequently lowering skin temperature. The cool shell of skin now acts as an insulating layer for the deeper core areas of the body; skin temperatures may drop nearly as low as that of the surrounding environment, while the body's core temperature remains at its normal 98.6° F (37° C). With a large temperature drop on the skin's surface, however, the sense of touch and pain is diminished. If cooling is continued, underlying muscles are affected and coordination is impeded. It becomes more difficult to strike a match, tie a cord, or handle a small object. Shivering begins early after exposure to cold, and becomes uncontrollable if exposure continues.

Signs of a reduced capacity to make judgments also appear rapidly. The victim becomes withdrawn or apathetic, or makes poor decisions. As the body's core drops below 95° F (35° C), the victim may become confused and sleepy and show further loss of coordination. Walking becomes difficult, and movements are stiff and awkward. Uncontrollable shivering may stop, and pulse and respiration may slow. As the core temperature approaches 80° F (30° C), the victim may become unconscious, and pulse and respiration will weaken or even stop. A cold heart is very sensitive. Unnecessary movement of an extremely cold victim may cause the heart to begin beating erratically or stop completely. A very cold motionless victim, without pulse and respiration, may be revived without permanent damage. The victim should never be considered dead until after warming. A good rule of thumb is: "No one is dead until warm and dead." The basic goal of first aid for hypothermia is to prevent further heat loss.

Unfortunately, the signs and symptoms of hypothermia do not always conform to the severity of the condition. One victim with a very low core temperature may remain conscious and rational, while another victim with little core cooling may act very confused and have great difficulty with coordination. The best sign of hypothermia is core temperature. While an oral temperature will not always give an accurate measure of core temperature (it should be lower than the core unless the victim has recently drunk or eaten warm food), it can be a guide to treatment.

MILD HYPOTHERMIA. For purposes of field treatment of hypothermia, the condition can be divided into mild and moderate-to-severe levels. Any victim with an oral temperature of 95° F (35° C) or less should be suspected to have moderate-to-severe hypothermia.

Signs and Symptoms of Mild Hypothermia

- Oral temperature down to 95° F (35° C)
- Complaints of cold
- Shivering
- Difficulty with using the hands
- Psychological withdrawal and apathy

FIRST AID FOR MILD HYPOTHERMIA

1. End exposure—get the victim out of the cold and wet.

2. Replace wet clothing with dry, or add insulation to clothing.

3. Place the victim in a warm environment; the victim should be able to return to normal temperature with little other intervention.

4. Offer warm liquids or food only if the victim is fully conscious and able to swallow food easily.

Signs and Symptoms of Moderate
or Severe Hypothermia

- Oral temperatures lower than 95° F (35° C)
- Lethargy, mental confusion, and refusal to recognize the problem
- Uncontrollable shivering
- Slurred speech
- Stumbling

MORE SEVERE SIGNS

- Unresponsiveness
- Decreased pulse and respiration
- Cessation of shivering
- Physical collapse

MODERATE-TO-SEVERE HYPOTHERMIA. If the victim remains cold for a number of hours, chemical changes begin to take place in the body, particularly in the limbs. On rewarming, these chemical changes may cause major problems for the victim, which could result in death. Severely hypothermic victims are best warmed in the hospital under controlled conditions. If the evacuation will be quick, protect the victim from further heat loss. End exposure to the cold and gently replace wet clothing.

If a severely hypothermic victim cannot be gotten to medical care within a few hours, rewarming should begin in the field. Begin attempts to rewarm a hypothermia victim found in the late afternoon or early evening, since rescue from the mountains to a hospital will not be completed until the next evening.

Prevention of Hypothermia

Prevention of hypothermia involves prevention of heat loss, termination of exposure, and early detection of signs of emerging illness.

PREVENTING HEAT LOSS. The following activities can be undertaken:

- Control evaporative heat loss by regulating clothing to prevent excessive sweating.
- Cover areas that are particularly sensitive to radiative heat loss: head, neck, and hands. Remember the old saying, "if your feet are cold put on a hat."
- Prevent convective heat loss by wearing layers of clothing, which will help to maintain the layer of warm air next to the body. Heat

is lost rapidly with the lightest breeze unless this layer is maintained.

- Prevent conductive heat loss by placing insulation between the body and cold objects. A sit pad can provide significant insulation between an individual's posterior and a cold rock or patch of snow. Wetting of clothes, particularly cotton, reduces their insulative ability greatly.
- Wear clothes that will maintain their insulative properties when wet, or will wick wetness away from the body. Cotton pants should not be the only clothing carried by the mountaineer.
- Prevent heat loss during breathing by covering the mouth and nose with wool or other insulative material. This will also help to reduce heat loss by prewarming the air that will enter the lungs.

TERMINATING EXPOSURE. If you cannot stay dry and warm under the existing conditions, terminate exposure by getting out of the wind and rain. Bivouac early before energy is exhausted and before coordination and judgment are impaired. Eat foods high in carbohydrates and sugars, which can be quickly converted to heat by the body. Avoid alcohol, which opens surface blood vessels resulting in a false sense of warmth but an actual loss of body heat. Keep continuously active to ensure adequate heat production.

FIRST AID FOR MODERATE OR SEVERE HYPOTHERMIA

First Aid if Victim WILL BE Evacuated Promptly

1. End exposure—cover the victim, rather than walking the victim into shelter.
2. Treat the victim very gently—clothing may have to be cut off to prevent unnecessary jostling or movement.
3. Do not allow the victim to exercise or move. Such movement may force cold blood present in the limbs into the core of the body, further decreasing core temperature.
4. Check the victim for other injury, including frostbite.

Further First Aid if the Victim WILL NOT BE Evacuated Promptly

5. Rewarming of the victim should focus on delivering warmth to the head, neck, armpits, and groin areas. Heat will most easily reach the core of the body from these regions. Warmth may be delivered by application of warm water-bottles, warmed blankets, or another warm body. Care should be taken not to burn the victim.
6. Offer warm food or liquid only when the victim seems fully conscious and has no difficulty in swallowing.

EARLY DETECTION. Any time a party is exposed to wind, cold, or wetness, carefully watch each individual for the symptoms of hypothermia. Treatment of early hypothermia is relatively simple compared to the efforts needed to deal with a severely ill individual. The victim may deny having any problems. BELIEVE THE SIGNS AND SYMPTOMS, NOT THE VICTIM.

Frostbite

One way in which the body protects itself on exposure to cold is to constrict surface blood vessels. The hands have the greatest skin area for their volume of any part of the body, and therefore cool very rapidly. The fingers, toes, ears, and nose, which protrude from the body, are quite susceptible to cooling and frostbite. If the temperature continues to drop, circulation will almost completely cease and frostbite will occur. The water in between cells freezes, and the water inside the cells moves out in response to chemical imbalances caused by the freezing. Tissues are injured physically from the expansion of the ice and by the resultant imbalances within each cell. The basic goal of first aid for frostbite is to prevent further areas of damage by additional freezing or refreezing of tissue.

SUPERFICIAL FROSTBITE. The signs and symptoms of frostbite vary in degree of severity and extent. Generally, frostbite can be divided into two categories: superficial and deep. In superficial frostbite, only small patches of surface tissue are affected, typically on the exposed areas of faces, noses, ears, and hands. In deep frostbite, deeper tissues and more extensive areas are frozen, which may involve the hands and feet and portions of legs and arms. Superficial frostbite is not as serious as deep frostbite, but it should be seen as a warning that deeper frostbite is a real risk if the condition of the victim is not improved.

DEEP FROSTBITE. Deep frostbite is a serious problem that can result in loss of tissue or an entire body part. Early recognition of frostbite and prevention of any further injury as a result of infection, trauma, or allowing the part to thaw and refreeze is essential if the loss of tissue is to be minimized.

Signs and Symptoms of Superficial Frostbite

SIGNS	SYMPTOMS
• Small patches of white or waxy skin • Patches are hard to the touch, underlying tissues are soft	• Pain may be felt early • The area may feel intensely cold or numb

FIRST AID FOR SUPERFICIAL FROSTBITE

1. Place a warm body part next to the frozen area, applying firm, steady pressure.

2. DO NOT RUB the area. Rubbing may cause damage to already injured skin.

3. Protect the area from further freezing.

Once a frozen part has thawed, the victim may become a litter case. The part will be extremely painful; travel on a thawed foot will be almost impossible. If a frozen part accidentally thaws and refreezes, greater tissue damage will occur. Loss of a hand or foot is much more likely in the case of thawing and refreezing.

Thawing should be undertaken ONLY if refreezing will not take place, and if the body part can be kept under sterile conditions. This will be almost impossible to maintain in the field. To thaw a frozen part: immerse the part in a water bath at 102° F (38.5° C) to 105° F (41° C). The bath must be kept at a constant temperature by the addition of warmed water. A thermometer is essential for monitoring the temperature of the water. Continue the thawing until the part is completely thawed, or "pink to the tip." The pink color indicates that circulation has been restored. A part that is severely damaged may not regain complete circulation. If the pink color does not return to the limb in a reasonable amount of time, remove the part from the bath. Encourage exercise of thawed toes or fingers during and after thawing. Once thawed, place the part on a sterile pad, placing small pieces of sterile gauze between toes and fingers. If hypothermia is present, delay thawing of the part until the hypothermia has been treated. Do not use hot water-bottles, heat lamps, or place the part near a hot stove, as excessive heat may cause further damage. Do not disturb blisters, since the possibility of infection is great. Take the victim to a hospital or other medical assistance.

Signs and Symptoms of Deep Frostbite

SIGNS	SYMPTOMS
• Skin is white, and may be waxy in appearance	• Pain may be felt as the part freezes
• The skin is hard to the touch, underlying tissues are solid	• The part will become numb and senseless
• Joint movement will be absent or restricted	• On thawing, the part will be very painful
• The area may be as small as part of a finger or involve a whole limb	

FIRST AID FOR DEEP FROSTBITE: IN THE FIELD

- KEEP THE FROZEN PART FROZEN.
- Prevent further injury: AVOID rubbing and further freezing of unaffected tissue.
- If the part has thawed, the part should NOT be allowed to refreeze or bear weight. A victim with thawed feet should be carried out.
- Give the victim plenty of fluids.
- Evacuate as soon as possible.

PREVENTING FROSTBITE. The following steps can be taken:

- Wear sufficient clothing to prevent injury. Mittens are better than gloves. Face masks may be necessary in strong, cold winds.
- Clothing should be loose enough to prevent constriction of blood vessels. Boots should not be tied tightly, and lacing should be checked frequently to ensure adequate circulation to the feet.
- An extra layer of socks should not be added to the feet if the boots will then become too tight and restrict circulation.
- If felt bootliners are worn, check to be sure that freezing and expansion of the felt has not impeded circulation to the feet.
- Do not touch metals as heat is conducted quickly away.
- Do not touch gasoline with the bare skin. The rapid evaporation of gasoline may quickly lead to frozen tissues.
- Exercise the toes and fingers to help maintain circulation.
- Observe the conditions of your partner's face, hands, and ears frequently for any indication of superficial frostbite.
- Avoid smoking before and during exposure.

Effects of Excessive Heat

The body reacts to an increase in temperature in two ways: by dilating the skin's blood vessels, allowing more blood to pass near the surface to be cooled; and by the evaporation of perspiration. Sweating results in the loss of water and electrolytes (salts). Elevated body temperature and the loss of too much electrolytes and water may result in a number of heat-related illnesses.

Heat Cramps and Fainting

Muscular cramps in the limbs or abdomen may result from a loss of water or electrolytes combined with physical exercise. Resting, massaging, and stretching the muscle may reduce the spasm. Give the victim plenty of water and avoid further strenuous exercise. Fainting in a hot environment may result from the pooling of blood in the legs. Victims usually recover

Signs and Symptoms of Heat Exhaustion

SIGNS	SYMPTOMS
• Pale skin color	• Nausea
• Sweating—usually profuse	• Weakness
• Skin temperature normal or slightly cool	• Dizziness
• Oral temperature normal or slightly elevated	• Thirst
	• Headache

quickly after collapse. Give the victim plenty of water or a slightly salty liquid. Flavored powders containing electrolytes added to water, usually marketed for athletes, may also be given.

Heat Exhaustion

Heat exhaustion occurs when the body's rate of heat gain is greater than the rate of heat loss. Heat exhaustion usually occurs during warm weather, but the weather need not be hot. Cross-country skiers can experience heat exhaustion if adequate water and electrolytes have not been consumed during the course of a hard day-trip. Thirst is not a reliable indicator of need for water, and will not occur until the body has lost about one quart. Dehydration is a major factor in the development of heat exhaustion.

Fluids should be given in small sips because the victim may be nauseated. Salted water may add to that discomfort. Flavoring the water may help to reduce the chance of vomiting. Once the victim has cooled down, replacement of electrolytes may be undertaken by giving bouillon or other salty foods.

Heat Stroke

Heat stroke is a life-threatening condition which may quickly lead to

FIRST AID FOR HEAT EXHAUSTION

1. Place the victim in a cool, shady environment.

2. Give the victim water in sips. (Electrolyte solutions may be used.)

3. Activity should not be resumed until the signs and symptoms are completely gone. Observe the victim for recurrence of heat exhaustion.

Signs and Symptoms of Heat Stroke

SIGNS	SYMPTOMS
• Irrational, confused, or combative behavior	• Weakness
• Pale, damp, relatively cool skin OR Red, dry, hot skin	• Irritability
	• Dizziness
• Oral temperature greater than 105° F (41° C)	• Headache

collapse and death. In heat stroke the body's internal temperature is usually above 105° F (41° C). Individuals resuming an active sport after a long period of inactivity, or exercising in a hot and humid environment to which they are not accustomed, may suffer from heat stroke. Their skin will initially appear pale, damp, and relatively cool, although their internal temperature is dangerously high. The most apparent sign of heat stroke for these victims is an irrational change in their behavior; they may become confused, irrational, or combative and aggressive.

In contrast, the most common urban victims of heat stroke are elderly, obese, or alcoholic. The skin of these individuals is usually red, hot, and dry to the touch. The common sign of all types of victims is the extremely high internal temperature. The goal of treatment for heat stroke is to quickly reduce body temperature.

PREVENTION OF HEAT-RELATED ILLNESSES. The following steps can be taken:

- Drink large amounts of water, even when thirst does not indicate a need. Water stops should be scheduled, even in cool weather or at high altitude.

FIRST AID FOR HEAT STROKE

1. DECREASE BODY TEMPERATURE IMMEDIATELY:
   a. remove or loosen tight clothing;
   b. place victim in cool, shady environment;
   c. cool the victim with cool cloths or cool water applied to the head, neck, armpits, and groin; vigorous fanning will help the cooling;
   d. if the victim is conscious, give water in sips.

2. The victim must be carried out and needs hospitalization

- Regulate activity to time of day, temperature, and condition of the party to avoid unnecessary exposure to heat stress.
- Taking salt tablets is NOT recommended.

PREVENTION OF HEAT INJURIES IS BASED IN ADEQUATE CONSUMPTION OF WATER AND ELECTROLYTES. Table salt should not be taken in large amounts unless water is freely available. The amount of electrolytes obtained in the usual diet is sufficient for most individuals even in the hottest weather. Some individuals may feel better in hot weather with a slight increase in table salt consumption. Hikers may wish to carry pretzels or some other salty snack to nibble while on the trail. Flavored powders containing electrolytes added to water may be used to replace electrolytes lost to sweat. Adequate consumption of water is the key to the prevention of heat-related illnesses.

Effects of High Altitude

A number of illnesses are related to rapid ascent to altitudes over 8,000 feet (2438 meters). Altitude illness may be a nuisance to the climber, or it may be a life-threatening problem if not treated quickly. Occasionally, altitudes of only 5,000 feet (1524 meters) may bring on mild symptoms for some people. Others will not be affected at much higher altitudes. The young, strong climber seems to be particularly susceptible to altitude problems. The healthy, well-conditioned climber is as frequently affected as the out-of-shape climber, and altitude problems may strike individuals already acclimated to altitude. Altitude illnesses strike unpredictably; climbers must not minimize early symptoms of illness which are similar to those of exhaustion.

Altitude illnesses seem to be related to decreased oxygen and air pressure, and their effects on blood and the brain. The illnesses are commonly divided into Acute Mountain Sickness, High Altitude Pulmonary

Signs and Symptoms of Acute Mountain Sickness

SIGNS	SYMPTOMS
• Difficulty with sleep	• Headache, mild to severe
• Unusual patterns of breathing, more obvious at night and during sleep	• Weakness and dull pain in muscles
• Fast, bounding pulse at rest	• Lack of appetite, nausea
• Vomiting	• Dizziness
• Puffiness in hands and face	• Shortness of breath
• Decreased and darker urine	

Edema, and High Altitude Cerebral Edema. The primary first aid goal for all altitude problems is descent to lower altitudes.

Acute Mountain Sickness

The signs and symptoms of Acute Mountain Sickness vary greatly in their severity. Symptoms may take a number of days to develop after the climber has reached altitude. Minor symptoms may disappear in a few hours or days if the climber remains at altitude. Any persistent symptom or any major symptom, such as severe headache or great difficulty with breathing during sleep, should be cause for undertaking the primary first aid—descent to lower altitude.

High Altitude Pulmonary Edema

Pulmonary edema is the leakage of fluid into the lungs, making breathing difficult. It is a serious condition which requires quick treatment —DESCENT, DESCENT, DESCENT!! The symptoms are related to the filling of the lungs with fluid, and are often accompanied by a great sense of anxiety as breathing becomes progressively more difficult. This condition may be seen as low as 8,000 feet (2438 meters), and seems to be associated with rapid ascent and immediate physical exertion upon arrival at altitude. The first cases were described as "skier's pneumonia," as they were found in lowland individuals who began skiing immediately after flying to resorts above 10,000 feet (3048 meters). Onset of symptoms may not be immediate, and may take several days to develop. Early symptoms may resemble mountain sickness. Any persistent cough, at rest or during exercise, may be an early indication of pulmonary edema. If allowed to proceed without descent, the victim will become unconscious and may have pink bubbles

---

FIRST AID FOR ACUTE MOUNTAIN SICKNESS

- Make a conscious effort to breathe deeply and regularly, or through pursed lips. If dizziness or nausea develops, stop rapid breathing.
- Slow down the pace of travel, use the "rest step."
- Increase the amount of fluids drunk. At high altitude, dehydration is a threat and seems to be related to mountain sickness.
- Aspirin may be taken for minor headache.
- Rest if symptoms make travel difficult.
- If symptoms are beyond a reasonable level of discomfort, descend to lower altitude.

Signs and Symptoms of High Altitude Pulmonary Edema

SIGNS	SYMPTOMS
• A dry cough at first, later producing watery sputum which may become pink	• Headache
	• Nausea and lack of appetite
• Gurgling sounds, as fluid increases in lungs	• Dizziness
	• Increasing anxiety
• Very rapid pulse, over 120/min	• Weakness and fatigue
• In later stages, the victim becomes incoherent, may have hallucinations	• Difficulty breathing
• In last stage, victim drops into coma, death in 6 to 12 hrs	

appear at the nose or mouth as more fluid enters the lungs. During the night, breathing may stop. Without descent, the victim may die.

Currently a device is being tested that, when worn over the mouth and nose, increases the amount of oxygen breathed and thereby mimics some effects of descent. This mask may become a part of first aid for pulmonary edema, although it is unlikely ever to become a substitute for descent.

High Altitude Cerebral Edema

Cerebral edema is a condition in which the brain swells within its bony case. This condition seems to take several days to develop, with twenty-four to forty-eight hours of mild mountain sickness followed by another twenty-four to forty-eight hours of increasingly severe symptoms before the emergence of specific signs and symptoms. Occasional cases have been reported as developing shortly after arrival at altitude. Signs and symptoms may include disorientation, confusion, and hallucinations.

Walking or other coordinated activities become difficult. A simple test for early cerebral edema is to ask the victim to follow a straight line walking toe-to-heel. If the victim loses balance and begins to fall over, cerebral edema must be suspected.

The victim may lie in a tent, not getting up to take meals, not speaking, not even going out to pass urine. If the condition is not treated, the victim will lapse into coma in twelve to twenty-four hours. Definitive treatment is descent. The party should not wait for rescue or other help if descent is at all possible. With any indication of possible cerebral edema, descent MUST be undertaken.

FIRST AID FOR HIGH ALTITUDE PULMONARY EDEMA

1. Descend.
2. Descend.
3. Descend to lower altitude at the first indication of pulmonary edema.
4. If descent is not possible, the victim must be carefully monitored for breathing difficulties, particularly at night.
5. Assist breathing as necessary.

PREVENTION OF ALTITUDE ILLNESSES. The following steps can be taken:

- Ascend to altitude in stages, allowing the body time to acclimate.
- Climb slowly. Above 10,000 feet (3048 meters) it is wise to allow one day per 1,000 feet (305 meters) of elevation gained for acclimatization.
- Once reaching altitude, rest is essential. Only light physical exercise should be performed for the first twenty-four hours.
- If climbing a number of summits, descend to the lowest possible level for sleep. "Climb high, sleep low."
- Consume sufficient water to prevent dehydration; you must drink much more than needed to slake thirst.
- Eat sufficient food to maintain energy levels.
- At the first sign of severe headache, persistent coughing, or mental confusion, descend to lower altitude.
- Acetazolamide, a prescription drug, has been shown to prevent symptoms of altitude illnesses. It should be used only if the individual has had repeated bouts of illness.

The Human Body Under Stress

This section has dealt with illnesses experienced from stresses placed on the human body. Heat, cold, and high altitude all require adaptations by the body to maintain normal levels of functioning. Adaptation requires energy, gained from food and water, aided by adequate rest and physical conditioning. If that energy is not available, the individual will become sick in some fashion. It is not surprising that many of the illnesses discussed in this section resemble fatigue at their onset, and that their symptoms are reduced by eating food and drinking water.

Heavy physical activity increases the body's need for energy and water.

An average adult requires approximately 5000 calories per day for heavy activity. To accomplish this, a conscientious intake of food should be maintained in small quantities every hour. Diets should contain large quantities of carbohydrates, which are quickly converted into glucose and carried into the bloodstream. But they should not be eaten to the exclusion of fatty foods and proteins. Fats and proteins take considerably longer to digest, but are important for providing long-term energy.

As the body exerts itself and heat builds, it perspires. During strenuous activity, particularly at high altitude, the amount of fluids lost through perspiration and evaporation of moisture from the lungs may be as much as five quarts or more per day. If a substantial amount of fluid is lost and not replaced, the body's chemical equilibrium is upset and illness is more likely to occur. Fluid intake for a twelve-hour day of moderate activity should be at least two quarts in temperate climates. Fluid intake for a longer climb or for more severe activity should be from two to five quarts. Enough water should be drunk to keep the urine clear and straw colored. The body CANNOT continue without adequate fluids, as it can without food, for more than a few hours or days.

The efficiency with which energy can be used by the body is related to physical conditioning and fatigue. The greater the level of physical conditioning, the greater efficiency with which food and water are used by the body. Consequently, greater physical conditioning is related to decreased susceptibility to illness such as hypothermia and frostbite. A fatigued climber is more likely to experience difficulties with heat or cold than a well-rested, well-fed climber. Prevention of many of the environmentally related illnesses is related to the body's ability to use food and water in an efficient manner to combat the stresses of heat, cold, and altitude. Adequate consumption of food and water, sufficient rest, and a good level of physical conditioning are essential components of prevention of environmentally related illness and enjoyment of the mountains.

SUDDEN MAJOR ILLNESS

Sudden major illness (such as heart attack) is relatively rare in the mountaineering setting. However, the ability to recognize and then aid a victim of a sudden illness can literally mean the difference between life and death.

Difficulty Breathing

Difficulty breathing, or "shortness of breath," is a symptom—the subjective sensation of not getting enough air. The victim may additionally have objective signs, such as a rapid breathing rate or speaking in short phrases only.

There are a variety of reasons for the sudden appearance of difficulty breathing, ranging from the unexpected worsening of some long-standing disease, such as asthma, to some totally new process occurring within the body. The most likely causes in the backcountry are an allergic reaction or a partial obstruction of the airway, as from a piece of fruit or cheese.

The victim of an acute asthma attack will usually have had one before, and know what is happening. Similarly, the victim of an allergic reaction may also be aware of having the existing medical condition known as "hypersensitivity." On the other hand, although the victim of a partial obstruction of the airway may be aware of what is happening, he or she may not be able to tell you: if the airway is blocked, the victim can't talk.

IMMEDIATE ACTION. Any person with major difficulty breathing should be evacuated as soon as possible, by self-evacuation when feasible. People who are having difficulty breathing are usually more comfortable sitting up. Victims of *asthma attacks* will benefit from a calm approach. First aid for an *allergic reaction* includes the application of constricting bands (if the victim has been stung or bitten) and an awareness of the possibility of the onset of shock. The first aid for an *obstructed airway* has been discussed in Chapter 2: if the victim is not moving air in or out, then start the abdominal thrusts.

Chest Pain

Chest pain is a subjective sensation, and can be described as "sharp," "squeezing," "crushing," "tightness," and so on.

The most common cause of chest pain is heart disease, but in a mountaineering setting it is more likely due to a chest injury (rib fracture). Other possible causes include a spontaneous collapsed lung, which occasionally occurs in young people who are exercising heavily.

Usually the victim of heart disease is aware of the problem, although many victims of a heart attack will deny the seriousness of the pain. The pain from a heart attack may radiate down the left arm, and be associated with an irregular pulse and cool, clammy skin. Some heart disease patients have *angina*, which is chest pain that comes on with exertion, cold, or emotional stress. Unlike heart attack, angina is generally relieved by rest, and rarely lasts more than ten minutes.

The pain from a spontaneous collapsed lung is usually sharp, confined to a small area, and is associated with coughing and difficulty breathing.

IMMEDIATE ACTION. Most victims with chest pain are more comfortable sitting up. The victim of a *heart attack* should be placed in a semireclining position and monitored closely for signs of shock or possible sudden cardiac arrest. If shock occurs, raise the victim's legs twelve to fourteen inches; if the heart stops, start CPR. Often the patient with heart disease will have medications that a physician has prescribed—you can assist him or her in taking them as necessary (but do not administer them on your own).

The victim of a *spontaneous collapsed lung* may be more comfortable lying, with the affected side down.

Any victim with serious chest pain needs to be evacuated as soon as possible, by self-evacuation when feasible.

Unconsciousness

Unconsciousness can result from either sudden illness, injury, or both together, and thus a thorough head-to-toe examination is important. Causes include: head injury, stroke, shock, epileptic seizure, diabetic emergency, asphyxia (oxygen deprivation), and heat stroke.

A *head injury* may be obvious from the appearance or history of what happened; a slow pulse may also be found. The *stroke* victim may initially have had a severe headache, and may have paralysis on one side. The victim in *shock* will have a fast pulse and cool, clammy skin. An *epileptic seizure,* or "convulsion," generally lasts about two minutes and is most often followed by about five minutes of unconsciousness. *Diabetic* patients often have medical identification bracelets. *Asphyxia* (oxygen deprivation) may be obvious—as in a drowning victim—or not—as in carbon monoxide poisoning (which can occur when cooking in a snow cave or tent without ventilation). *Heat stroke* victims may have hot, red skin.

IMMEDIATE ACTION. The number-one priority with an unconscious victim is to be sure that the AIRWAY is open. Once the airway is assured, do the head-to-toe exam. Remember that all unconscious injury victims are assumed to have a neck injury until proven otherwise, so immobilize the spine. The unconscious uninjured victim can be positioned on the side, to help maintain an open airway. All unconscious victims will need to be evacuated as soon as possible. Monitor the victim's vital signs frequently.

Head injury, shock, and heat stroke have been discussed previously in this book. First aid for oxygen deprivation (*asphyxia*) consists of providing good air and artificial respiration when necessary.

First aid for a *diabetic emergency* actually consists of doing something before the victim becomes unconscious. The diabetic patient can have problems when there is an imbalance between food intake, exercise, and insulin shots. Two conditions can result: high blood sugar or low blood sugar. High blood sugar is characterized by a gradual onset and dry, red skin. Low blood sugar is characterized by rapid onset and pale, moist skin. The diabetic may recognize the signs and know what to do; but, if the victim is confused or disoriented, first aid always consists of giving the victim sugar. If the victim becomes unconscious, sugar such as hard candy or chocolate can be placed inside the cheek, in small amounts, repeatedly.

EYE CARE. If the victim is unconscious for more than one hour, some special procedures need to be done to protect the eyes. Keep the eyelids closed to slow drying of the surface of the eye and to prevent scratching of the eyeball.

The unconscious victim with contact lenses will need to have the contacts removed. When the eyes are kept closed continuously, without blinking, for long periods of time, the moisture normally present begins to disappear. Without moisture, less oxygen can get to the surface of the eye, and damage can result. The contact lens may also adhere to the surface of the eye as it dries. Even soft contact lenses, which under normal circumstances readily allow moisture and oxygen to pass through, can dry out and adhere to the surface.

Soft contact lenses are removed by grasping the lens in a pinching motion between the thumb and forefinger. Hard contact lenses can be removed by using a small, specially designed suction device, and some lens wearers carry this as part of their personal first aid kit. Another method is to separate the eyelids and use the index finger to pull outward from the outer edge of the eye. This will cause a blinking-like motion of the eyelid, which should pop up the hard lens. The contact can then be lifted off the eyeball.

Allergic Reactions

Allergic reactions occur when the body reacts in a self-destructive fashion to the presence of a foreign substance. Allergic reactions kill twice as many people each year as snakebites.

Foreign substances can enter the body in a number of different ways: with an insect bite or sting, as from a wasp or a bee; or through inhalation, as of pollen; or in food, such as nuts. The seriousness of an allergic reaction can vary from mild symptoms of itching and burning to severe anaphylactic shock. It is difficult to predict which victims of allergic reaction will progress to severe shock.

Most people with severe allergies are aware of this problem, and they often wear medical identification bracelets. The victim having an allergic reaction may first be aware of a generalized warmth and itching, particularly of the hands and feet. The next symptom may be difficulty breathing, and signs such as a rash, hives, and wheezing may appear. Swelling of the lips, tongue, eyelids, and hands may follow. The signs of shock (rapid, weak pulse; pale, cool, clammy skin) will be late findings, and signify a poor prognosis in a mountaineering setting.

IMMEDIATE ACTION. The victim of an allergic reaction should be evacuated as soon as possible, primarily because of the difficulty in predicting whether the condition will worsen. Many people with known allergies carry small kits with them, which contain syringes of medications such as adrenaline and/or diphenhydramine (Benadryl). (Some people now carry adrenaline inhalers.) If the victim has prescribed medications, it is appropriate to assist the person in taking them.

MINOR MISERIES

Blisters

Blisters are caused by friction from rubbing, which can occur when boots are too large (or too small) or are laced too loosely, or when socks are wrinkled. *Downhill blisters* occur on the toes when the foot slides forward in the boot, and *uphill blisters* are found on the heel.

PREVENT FURTHER INJURY. Remove the boot and sock at the first sign of a hot spot, and protect any reddened area by covering with moleskin (or tape or molefoam). Be sure that it extends well beyond the reddened area. If a blister has already formed, keep pressure off it by applying a doughnut-shaped piece of moleskin or molefoam.

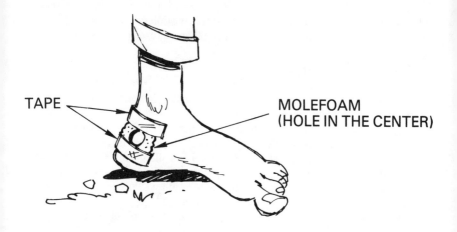

TAPE

MOLEFOAM
(HOLE IN THE CENTER)

PREVENT INFECTION. Blisters should not be opened unless absolutely necessary. If it must be done, wash the area with soap and water, and insert a needle (sterilized with a match or rubbing alcohol) at the edge of the blister. Gently press out the fluid and apply a sterile dressing.

If the blister has already broken, it should be washed and dressed in the same manner as any open wound.

PREVENTION OF BLISTERS. The best prevention of blisters is to wear properly fitting boots, well broken in, with two pairs of socks. Many people put adhesive tape or moleskin over areas that blister easily before hiking. Some people find that benzoin, applied repeatedly over a period of weeks, can toughen the skin.

Headache

Headache in the mountains can result from dehydration, eye strain from inadequate protection from the sun, or tension in the neck muscles. It can also result from lack of sleep, or be related to drinking alcohol (habits not unknown to climbers). Less often, it is an early sign of a more serious problem, such as heat exhaustion or acute mountain sickness. In any cause of headache, the source of the trouble should be sought and first aid given as appropriate. Aspirin may relieve the immediate pain.

Fainting

Fainting is caused by a temporary lessening of blood flow to the brain, generally from pooling in the legs. It can result from a wide variety of processes, including: prolonged standing, especially in the heat; sudden standing after resting; or less often, from fright (such as upon encountering a Sasquatch). Unconsciousness that lasts for more than three minutes is not considered fainting. First aid for fainting consists of positioning the victim flat, with lower legs raised. First aid for heat illness may also be indicated.

Diarrhea and *Giardia*

Although the clear mountain stream is likely free of the pollution caused by "civilization," it may well not be free of illness-causing bacteria or parasites. The United States Forest Service and Park Service are currently advising backcountry travelers to treat their water before drinking it to prevent infection with the parasite Giardia. Giardiasis is the number one parasite disease in the United States, and it affects some ten to twenty percent of the world's population. A trapping study of wild animals in Washington State found Giardia in nineteen percent of beavers and forty three percent of muskrats. Outbreaks have been reported from New England to California.

Giardia is transmitted both by drinking contaminated water and by direct person-to-person contact. Giardia cysts are too small to be seen, and even the clearest of streams can harbor thousands of cysts. Water can be contaminated by infected animals or infected people, underscoring the need for backcountry sanitation: bury your wastes away from streams, and wash your hands before preparing food.

If a person becomes infected, one of three things can happen. *Acute infection* is marked by diarrhea lasting ten days or more, foul-smelling stools and gas, fatigue, and abdominal distension. *Chronic infection* is marked by intermittent episodes of mushy, foul-smelling stools, abdominal pain and distension, gas, loss of appetite, weight loss, and fatigue. *Asymptomatic infection* means no symptoms are noticed by the infected person, but Giardia is present in the intestines. These people are carriers of infection, who can unknowingly infect others.

Symptoms of giardiasis, if they develop, occur seven to ten days after infection. First aid for diarrhea is limited to replacing the lost fluid. A balanced solution of salts and sugar, such as Gatorade or ERG, is best. Not all diarrhea is caused by Giardia (food preparation with dirty hands can also transmit bacteria); consultation with a physician may be required for an accurate diagnosis.

Because the consequences of infection are so unpleasant, the best approach is prevention. You can choose not to drink the water (and carry water from home), or treat it to kill the bacteria. Water treatment involves either boiling the water or using chemicals. Although some people object to the taste of the chemicals, it may not be practical to boil all water on all trips.

Chemical water treatment methods include the use of liquid disinfectants (such as chlorine bleach or povidone iodine), commercial disinfectant tablets, and the use of iodine crystals in saturated solution. Although the iodine crystal method is probably the most effective and least expensive, it is not the safest. Considerable caution must be used to avoid pouring crystals into the drinking water. Filtration devices, newly available in outdoor equipment stores, are still unproven.

RESPONDING TO THE EMOTIONALLY UPSET VICTIM

A victim's emotional response to an injury is an important factor in first aid. A positive attitude and will-to-survive can greatly help the victim and the rescuers deal with the stressful and frightening experience of an accident. Left unattended, emotional upset can result in the obstruction of first aid efforts, and can cause rescuers themselves to become upset. A few basic ideas can guide the first aider's response to the upset victim.

The rescuer's response will influence the victim's response. A calm, quiet approach by the rescuer will frequently lead to a similar response by the victim. Speak softly and slowly. Discuss injuries in terms that are not upsetting ("you have some bleeding" rather than "my goodness, it's gushing"). Keep the confusion of the accident scene to a minimum. It is better for one rescuer to talk with a victim than to have several rescuers asking multiple questions all at the same time, as this can only lead to confusion.

The rescuer must also build and maintain a sense of credibility with the victim. Respond truthfully to the victim, and do not give false reassurances. Telling the victim everything is "all right" when it is clearly not all right may indicate that the rescuer is not very bright or not to be trusted. Rescuers must be aware of their own feelings and reactions to an accident in order to give their best care. Comments of "you shouldn't feel that way" or "snap out of it" represent what the rescuer wishes. Such comments will not help the victim, nor will argument and denial of the realities of the situation. Treat the victim as you would wish to be treated, with honesty and concern.

The range of response to an injury may be wide. The victim may be very quiet and slow to respond to questions, or be very excited and unable to sit still. A frequent reaction is denial, a statement that a serious injury has not occurred. It is very frightening to admit that you cannot move your legs or that the pain in your forearm means a broken bone. Victims frequently will experience anger about the injury, panic that rescue will come too late, and general anxiety about what will happen next, and whether they will be able to get back to work on Monday. Some victims may experience waves of grief, and others may become very aggressive in response to the incident. All these feelings are normal reactions to an accident. Individuals respond in different ways. Not everyone can be expected to show the same set of feelings or the same tolerance to pain or injury. Feelings may change rapidly during the course of a rescue. Your companions may have similar difficulties in dealing with their own feelings generated by the accident scene. It is important to recognize these feelings and to help the victim (and the rescuers) cope with the confusion and fright of an accident.

There are several basic things a rescuer can do to help the victim deal with upsetting emotions:

GIVE INFORMATION. Introduce yourself and let the victim know what is going to be done. Respond to questions with honest answers. Share plans for further care with the victim.

LISTEN TO THE VICTIM. Let the victim talk about his or her fears and feelings. The rescuer may need to help the victim discuss feelings. Ask, "what are you thinking, how are you doing?" The rescuer may not agree with those feelings, but those feelings should be respected. Reassurances should come only after feelings have been accepted by the rescuer. Don't say, "You shouldn't be afraid." It is better to say "I can understand that you are very scared right now, but we will try to help you through this."

STAY WITH THE VICTIM. Do not leave a victim alone if at all possible. One rescuer should be assigned to supervise a victim. If there are more victims than rescuers, assign a rescuer to several victims closely grouped together. If a victim is very anxious or gets in the way, a rescuer may need to take the victim to an isolated location.

USE TOUCH. Holding a victim's hand or putting an arm around his or her shoulder can be very comforting. Holding a victim by the elbow may be helpful in moving the victim out of harm's way. If the victim does not want to be touched, that wish must be respected. Physical restraint is almost never necessary, and may result in injury to the rescuer if the victim is violent. Use of physical force is never acceptable, unless it is necessary to prevent injury to yourself or other victims.

DIRECT THE VICTIM'S THOUGHT. Asking the victim for information about the incident, involving the victim in making plans for treatment, or discussing details of life "back in the city" can help the victim to engage in constructive thought and to stop reviewing the ugly details of the accident. While directing the victim's thoughts can be helpful, the rescuer must be willing to listen to the victim's concerns and feelings.

DIRECT THE VICTIM'S ACTIVITY. If the victim is able to help, having the victim set up a tent, prepare food, or engage in any meaningful activity can help to calm the victim. The victim will begin to feel that his or her efforts are contributing to the solution of the problem.

PROVIDE COMFORT. Food, drink, warmth, and protection from further injury does much to help the upset victim. A warm cup of tea is very calming.

Upset feelings cannot be "cured," but the victim and rescuers can be helped to cope with feelings and their behavior can be directed to helpful activities. A few techniques can be very helpful in managing a stressful situation: give information, listen to the victim's fears and concerns, stay with the victim, use touch for comfort, direct the victim's thought and action towards positive activities, and provide the physical comforts of food, drink, and warmth.

Chapter 4: Short Distance Transfer and Evacuation Techniques

SHORT DISTANCE TRANSFER

Short distance transfer may be needed to move a victim off the snow, out of the rain, or into a tent. Such transfers can improve the comfort of a victim of a mountaineering accident. More importantly, moving the victim may be essential to first aid treatment and well being. For the seriously injured victim the LEAST amount of movement is probably the best. More harm can be done through improper transfer than through any other measure associated with first aid. Transfer of a victim should be done only when absolutely necessary and with a great deal of care and forethought.

In moving a victim, the following procedures must be observed:

- The airway must be open and serious bleeding stopped.
- Transfer should be undertaken only after initial pain and fear have subsided.
- Plan moves so that the victim must be moved only once.
- Prepare any insulating materials or shelter before the victim is moved.
- The transfer process should be rehearsed carefully, using a rescuer as practice subject. Directions for the transfer should be practiced.
- The rescuer supporting the head is the leader of the transfer. Other rescuers should follow the movement and direction of the leader precisely.
- Protection of the victim's entire body must be assured during the move. The body should be kept in a straight line.
- A "scout," a rescuer not holding onto the victim, may be appointed to help the rescuers avoid obstacles and travel over rough terrain.

Methods for the transfer of victims are carefully covered in standard first aid texts. The transfer methods are easily learned, but must be practiced before being used on a victim. Participation in a standard first aid class will aid in gaining these skills. The ability to use movement techniques correctly is of particular concern in the mountains because of the possibility of back, head, and neck injuries due to falls.

Transfer of a victim with a suspected back or neck injury

A victim with a suspected back or neck injury should be moved ONLY on a rigid backboard or litter. A rigid litter or board cannot be made from the materials typically at hand in a mountaineering situation, and its use usually requires advanced first aid training. Until a rigid litter can be brought to the scene of the accident, it is best to leave the victim as found, putting a shelter up around the victim rather than attempting to move the victim into shelter.

If the victim must be moved to allow placement of insulation between the victim and the ground, or must be transferred a short distance, the following techniques may be used. At all times during the movement, the victim's head and back must be kept in straight alignment. Once the move has ended, the head must be supported in a rescuer's grasp until it is secured with sandbags. This technique can be modified for use with victims found in other positions.

LOG-ROLL OF A VICTIM ONTO INSULATION: LYING ON THE BACK

1. The leader of the move assumes a position directly behind the victim's head. The rescuer's hands are positioned with fingers placed supporting the back of the head and the jaw, typically with the palms of the hands covering the ears. This may be modified due to the size of the rescuer's hands compared to the victim's head, or the position of the victim. The intent is to prevent motion of the victim's head relative to the rest of the body.
2. If necessary, the victim's head and neck may be moved gently and slowly to form a straight line with the back. If there is ANY resistance to the movement, or the victim experiences ANY pain, the movement must STOP IMMEDIATELY, and the head and neck be left in their present position.
3. The other rescuers assume positions on one side of the victim, kneeling on both knees. One rescuer is placed near the shoulders, the second at the hips, and a third at the knees.
4. The insulation material is placed on the far side of the victim, ready to move under the victim. The side of the material next to the victim may be rolled under itself, so that after the victim has been placed on the insulation the rolled edged may be gently unrolled.
5. The victim's arm on the same side as the rescuers is lifted up and out of the way of the roll, with support given to the shoulder so that the back and spine are moved as little as possible.
6. The rescuer at the shoulders holds the victim's other arm or

secures the arm by putting the victim's hand in a pocket or waistband.

7. The rescuer at the shoulders places one hand under the victim's far shoulder and the middle of the trunk. The rescuer at the hips places one hand at the top of the hips and the second midthigh. The rescuer at the knees places one hand under the knees, and the other cradling the ankles.

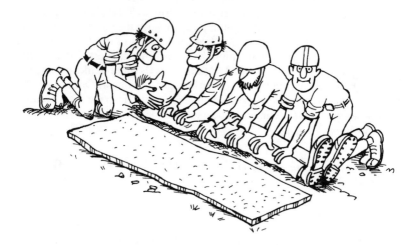

8. The leader calls "Prepare to roll," and when all are ready, "Roll": the victim is slowly rolled towards the rescuers' knees. The rescuer at the hips moves the insulation material under the victim.

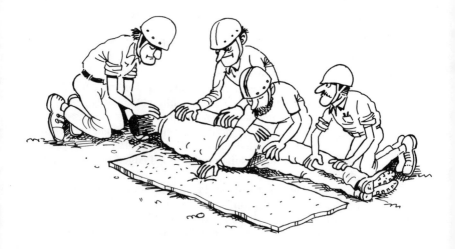

9. The leader calls "Prepare to lower," and then "Lower": the victim is rolled onto the material.
10. The rescuer at the victim's head remains in place until the head is secured with sandbags.

LOG-ROLL AND FOUR-PERSON-CARRY FOR SHORT-DISTANCE TRANSFER

1. The leader of the move assumes a position directly behind the victim's head. Hands are placed on either side of the head as in step one of the log-roll.
2. If necessary, the victim's head and neck may be moved gently and slowly to form a straight line with the back. If there is ANY resistance to the movement, or the victim experiences ANY pain, the movement must STOP IMMEDIATELY, and the head and neck be left in their present position.
3. The other rescuers assume positions on one side of the victim, kneeling on one knee. One rescuer is placed near the shoulders, the second at the hips, and a third at the knees.
4. The victim's arms are secured by gently tying them at the wrist or placing the hands in the waistband.
5. The rescuer at the shoulders gently moves one hand under the victim's shoulder and the other hand under the middle of the trunk.
6. The rescuer at the hips places one hand under the hips and the second below the thighs.
7. The rescuer at the knees places one hand under the knees, and the other cradling the ankles.
8. At the leader's calls "Prepare to lift," and "Lift," the victim is slowly lifted onto the rescuers' knees.

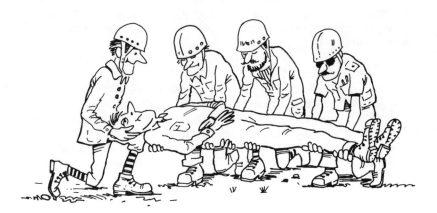

91

9. At the leader's calls "Prepare to stand," and "Stand," the rescuers stand erect.
10. Any further motion is directed by the leader.
11. Lowering the victim is the reverse of the procedure.

EVACUATION TECHNIQUES

Self-Evacuation

Most parties are not strong enough or well equipped enough to safely evacuate a seriously injured person. Frequently persons with relatively minor injuries can, with patience and care, be safely evacuated even by a small party. The leader, when deciding if self-evacuation is possible, must consider the extent of the injuries, the type of terrain to be covered, and the strength of other party members. The leader must also consider what will happen if the party starts to self-evacuate and is unable to continue. Will there be a safe place to stop? Several things are necessary to a successful self-evacuation.

The victim must be willing to help and must understand how to aid in the self-evacuation. All injuries must be treated prior to starting out. One person should accompany the victim at all times. He or she can provide both encouragement and physical assistance when needed. This person will also need to monitor the victim's condition and the safety of the evacuation procedures.

Each section of the evacuation route should be checked prior to attempting to navigate it with the victim. The other party members will have to travel the route at least two or even three times. Ways around obstacles need to be found prior to the arrival of the injured person, so that he or she does not have to backtrack or cross unnecessarily difficult areas. An apparently quicker more direct route might require the use of more balance or climbing techniques than the victim is capable of doing. A slight uphill section, barely noticed under normal conditions, may be an insurmountable barrier to the injured person.

Sending Out For Help

How quickly help will arrive, and how adequate it will be, depends on the kind of information sent out and the messenger's ability to deliver that information. Whenever possible, at least two people should be sent for help. They should never be sent until adequate information about the victim is available, the accident site is under control, and it is certain that their help will not be needed. The people sent should be stronger members of the party not only in terms of physical strength, but also in terms of experience and judgment. They must be able to get themselves out safely and deliver their message clearly and completely to the appropriate authorities. The messengers may also be asked to serve as guides back to the accident site.

The messengers should take the following information:

- Name, age, address, phone number of victim, who should be notified, and their relationship to the victim
- Where, when, and how the accident occurred
- The number of persons injured or ill, and the nature and seriousness of the injuries
- The first aid administered, the condition of the victim, including pulse, respiration and other vital signs from the initial exam and at the time the messengers left the party
- How many people and what equipment, including both first aid supplies and general equipment, are still at the scene, along with the party's condition and level of experience
- What equipment is needed — a rigid litter, food, water, shelter, etc.
- The party's EXACT LOCATION, and whether they will wait at the scene or will move to safer or more readily accessible ground
- Distance from the road and type of terrain: glacier, rock, or trail; be sure to include special information about local conditions, e.g.: "the last half mile of trail is covered with hard snow and is very steep"
- Local weather conditions, e.g.: is the accident site above the clouds, or is it very cloudy or windy?
- Method of evacuation necessary: carrying by rigid litter, sliding on snow, or lowering down steep cliffs
- The names and addresses of all members in the party, and whom to notify

Since it is impossible to remember all the information required, a written report must be carried out. A tear-out first aid report form is provided at the end of this book. The messengers will also need car keys and coins for the telephone.

The persons going for help should clearly mark the route. Brightly colored plastic surveyor's tape may be used. Any turn of the route or place where it leaves the trail should be especially well marked. In addition to the route, the location of the accident should be marked on a topographic map and brought out by the messengers.

Once the messengers reach a telephone, the proper agency must be notified of the accident. Which agency has jurisdiction depends on the location of the accident. In national parks the messengers should contact a ranger. Outside of the national parks, the responsible agency for rescues is usually the sheriff or state police department, and in Canada it is the Royal Canadian Mounted Police. Even when the proper agency has been contacted, the person on the telephone may not be familiar with rescue procedures or be uncertain if the accident is within their jurisdiction. The messengers must be persistent and patient in communicating the accident information to ensure that it does reach the person responsible for the agency's rescue response. The messengers need to remain at the telephone and be available if further information is needed. Rescue leaders may want to speak with the messengers or they may even ask the messengers to return to the accident site.

Increasingly, mountaineers are carrying small radios which enable rapid contact of outside help. Before attempting to contact outside help, the above information should be obtained, just as if messengers were going to carry it out. The use of radios can greatly reduce the time needed to request help.

Helicopter Rescue

The helicopter has revolutionized mountain rescue. It has evacuated injured from cliffs and glaciers directly to hospitals quickly and efficiently, when by ground it would have taken days of rough, exhausting travel. The helicopter is not, however, the "magic machine" some people think it to be. The weather may be such that a helicopter cannot respond. It may be clear where you are, but fogged in at the takeoff point. There may not be any helicopter available or you may be too far from its base or the closest fuel supply. Operations in the mountains are also very hazardous to both the pilot and the machine, and the costs of helicopter operations are very high. Never assume that a helicopter can come to your rescue.

CHOOSING A LANDING SITE. When requesting outside help, the party should choose a possible helicopter landing site and send out information on that site. The landing site should ideally be approachable from all sides for landings and takeoffs—a flat-topped ridge, for example. If a ridge is not close by, then choose a relatively flat area. The higher the elevation, the less load a helicopter can carry, and the more important a gradual climb becomes. A vertical takeoff is very demanding on the aircraft even at sea level, and may actually be impossible in the mountains.

PREPARING THE LANDING SITE. The landing site should be prepared prior to the arrival of the helicopter. The landing site should be made as level as possible. Mark the landing area with colored tape or other brightly colored objects. SECURELY ANCHOR ALL OBJECTS in the immediate area. Wind from the rotor can approach 60 to 120 miles per hour. Loose materials such as groundcloths, sleeping bags, or clothing can easily be blown upward into the rotor blades and cause serious problems. If the landing site is on soft snow, pack the site as much as possible to prevent blowing snow that could obstruct the pilot's vision.

PREPARING THE VICTIM. Prior to the arrival of the helicopter, the victim should be prepared for helicopter travel. Helicopters have limited fuel and cannot wait around very long while the victim is readied. Explain to the victim what you are doing and that when the helicopter arrives there will be a

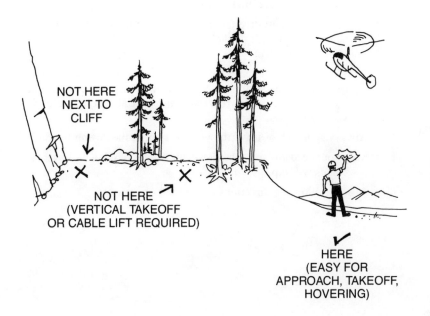

NOT HERE
NEXT TO
CLIFF

NOT HERE
(VERTICAL TAKEOFF
OR CABLE LIFT REQUIRED)

HERE
(EASY FOR
APPROACH, TAKEOFF,
HOVERING)

lot of noise and wind. Tie the victim's hands together if he or she is unconscious or semiconscious. Eye, ear, and head protection should be put on the victim. Any gear going with the victim should be placed in packs or stuff sacks. Be sure not to send out equipment such as ropes or clothing that may be needed later. Make sure that there are no loose straps or clothing. Attach in an obvious but very secure place the first aid record of the victim's injuries and first aid treatment given.

APPROACH AND LANDING. Brightly colored objects and arm-waving people are barely visible from the air. Consequently, when the helicopter approaches the area a signal with a smoke flare or a mirror can greatly speed up the pilot's locating the landing site. Once the helicopter is close, indicate wind direction using streamers of plastic surveyor's tape or a pair of ripstop nylon rain pants. If none of these is available, a party member can stand with arms extended toward the landing site, which indicates: "land here, my back is to the wind."

The following basic rules must be followed when the helicopter arrives:

- All people in the landing area should have eye protection and hardhats should be worn, if available. Dirt and other materials will be blown about the area when the helicopter lands.

- If the helicopter lowers a cable with a message, radio, or litter, allow it to touch ground first to dissipate static electricity.

- Stay at least seventy-five feet away from the helicopter when it is landing. Approach the helicopter only after signaled to by the pilot or crew chief.

- ALWAYS approach or leave the helicopter from the front so the pilot can see you at all times. NEVER go around the back of the helicopter, because the rear rotor blades are almost invisible and very dangerous.

- Always approach or leave the helicopter from the downhill side.

- Keep your head low since the slower the rotor is moving the lower the blades will dip.

- Always follow the directions of the pilot or crew.

Chapter 5: Making a Plan and Carrying It Out

STEP 6: PLAN WHAT TO DO

In previous sections discussion has focused on identifying types of injuries and providing methods of treating those injuries. Except for meeting the urgent first aid needs of impaired breathing and severe bleeding, there is no need to rush. It is better to stop and plan carefully what will be done and in what order. Planning can prevent moving the injured person unnecessarily or getting halfway through a treatment and having to undo it so that another part of the needed treatment can be done. The plan of care also extends beyond the immediate first aid needs of the victim to include deciding on means of evacuation and what roles party members will play. Although the final plan is the responsibility of the leader, information should be obtained from other members of the party about first aid needs and party resources. The leader may also discuss with party members ideas that they have about taking care of the first aid needs of the victims.

Establish Priorities

When planning care, a priority list of treatment needs should be established:

- *Are some victims more seriously injured than others?* Party resources may need to be focused on the most seriously injured in order that they may survive. Less seriously injured victims may get only a small part of the available help because they can survive with less assistance. Alternatively, if treatment needs of one victim are beyond the capacity of the party, then the party's resources should be directed toward caring for victims with injuries where they have a chance of success.

- *Which are the injuries that will cause the most harm if left unattended?* A broken leg may be painful and look bad, but it is not as hazardous to the victim's survival as being left lying on cold, wet ground.

- *Can treatment of one problem assist in the treatment of another problem?* For example, when moving the victim onto insulation, he or she can also be placed onto the ties needed for splinting. Making a priority list will help ensure that all treatment needs are met and that equipment and party members are used to their best advantage.

Deciding to Evacuate

After establishing a priority list for meeting the first aid needs of the victim, the leader must consider what will need to be done to keep the party safe and ensure that the injured can get to appropriate treatment. One of the most difficult questions that must be answered is how the injured person will get to outside help. Will the party self-evacuate or request outside help? Several conditions must be considered prior to making this decision:

- *What is the extent of the victim's injuries?* A minor injury may slow the party down, but given enough time the victim will be able to walk out. However, several relatively minor injuries or a severe injury may require more help than the party can provide.

- *What is the terrain that must be crossed?* A person with a broken wrist may be able to walk down a trail easily but have difficulty scrambling across a boulder field.

- *What is the weather?* Walking across an alpine slope in bright sunshine is much easier than trying to cross the same slope in wind, rain, and fog.

- *How far is it to the trailhead?* An injured person may be able to walk a mile or two, but not five or ten miles.

- *What is the party strength?* Party strength includes not only the number of people but also their condition, experience, and the equipment they have to use. A tired or inexperienced party may be unable to accomplish a self-evacuation.

- *What equipment is available?* Plan to use the victim's equipment first.

- *How much outside help is available and how long will it take to reach the accident scene?* In the mountains, outside help is usually six to twenty-four hours away. Even a slowly moving victim may be able to get out to help faster than help can get in.

The decision may not be a simple choice of self-evacuation versus requesting outside evacuation help, but a combination of the two types of evacuation. A party may move the victim a short distance to a safer or more comfortable location. They may self-evacuate to the point at which technical rescue techniques beyond the party's capacity are required. The party may move slowly down the trail toward the rescuers, thereby saving time.

STEP 7: CARRY OUT THE PLAN

After a complete examination of the entire accident situation and planning a course of action, the party is ready to carry out its plans. The leader needs to ensure that all aspects of the first aid care are done. Minor injuries should not be overlooked in the press of caring for major injuries.

Attention must also be given to how well the plan is working. Is the victim's condition improving or getting worse? Does the party have the abilities and resources to carry out the present plan? Is the party getting weaker, are party members becoming hypothermic? Is the party getting stronger and more confident as they realize they can handle the situation? Are there changes in terrain or weather that make the plan unworkable or inadequate? Constant evaluation of the plan must be made and changes made as needed.

Victim Monitoring

After the plan has been developed, a person should be assigned to continue monitoring and recording the victim's condition. Recording both the victim's vital signs and treatment given is essential in determining how well the plan is being carried out and how well the treatment is working. As part of the ongoing monitoring, vital signs need to be taken at regular intervals by the victim monitor.

The "victim monitor" is someone who stays with the victim constantly, someone who provides ever-present-contact. Every victim in the mountaineering setting will be anxious about what is happening, and it is the function of the victim monitor to stay by the side of the victim to provide reassurance and listen to his or her concerns. It is necessary to have the task of victim monitor assigned to a specific individual, because other members of the party may be doing something else, such as caring for another victim or having a conference about setting priorities. Monitoring of the victim is continued until the victim's care is assumed by a more advanced level of care provider.

Altering the Plan

Whatever the plan of action, both the leader and other party members will have to work together to carry out the plan successfully. The party will need to monitor the victim's condition and response to treatment. The party must not only work hard to carry out the plan, but also be willing to make changes in the plan if it is not working or if conditions change. Above all, in trying to perform first aid and/or rescue in a wilderness setting the people involved must keep open minds and think about what is needed and the alternatives that are available to take care of those needs.

Even with the best care that can be given, the injuries the victim has sustained may result in death. The death of a victim can be very frightening to the first aiders, causing them to feel insecure or afraid for their own lives. Some may feel guilt or remorse for their inability to save the person's life. If the victim dies, the leader will need to alter the focus from treating the victim to caring for party members. Directing each individual to constructive tasks of rescuing and caring for each other may be the most important task of the leader in the event of a death.

CONCLUSION

An accident scene is an extremely confused place. It is very difficult to sort through the things that can be done, to identify those which must be done, and then to accomplish them in proper order. Following the Seven Steps for First Aid Response can help guide the party members through the numerous tasks involved in performing first aid in a mountaineering environment. Like rock climbing or skiing, it DOES take practice to become proficient. Planning and mentally rehearsing actions in the event of an accident may be adequate practice for some. First aid courses with practical instruction in responding to mountaineering accidents are important to round out training.

Tremendous problems exist in the event of an accident in the backcountry far from medical care. Awareness of these problems may lead to a better sense of judgment and stimulate a conscientious effort to prevent injuries. Prevention includes knowing the causes of injuries and illness, planning one's own activities, and helping others to be aware of their own responsibilities for injury prevention. All who venture into the mountains have a responsibility to possess a working knowledge of how to respond to an accident situation. They have an even greater responsibility to help prevent avoidable injuries in the out-of-doors.

ABOUT THE AUTHORS

Martha J. Lentz, Ph.D., RN, is a faculty member of the University of Washington School of Nursing. She has worked in both orthopedic and emergency nursing. Lentz has been active in the Mountaineering Oriented First Aid program for the past ten years as an instructor and evaluator. An active climber, she is a graduate of The Mountaineers basic and intermediate climbing courses. As a member of the Seattle Mountain Rescue Council, she continues to participate in mountain rescue operations.

Steven C. Macdonald, M.P.H., EMT, is research consultant in the Division of Research in Medical Education, University of Washington School of Medicine. He is also chairperson of the Injury Control and Emergency Health Services Forum, American Public Health Association. He worked in the City of Boston Emergency Medical Service for five years prior to moving to Seattle for his graduate training in public health. Macdonald has been active as an instructor and evaluator in the Mountaineering Oriented First Aid program for the past six years, and edited The Mountaineers First Aid Committee newsletter, *First Aid Notes*, for two years. He is a graduate of The Mountaineers alpine scramble, winter travel, and basic climbing courses.

Jan Carline, Ph.D., has been involved with The Mountaineers First Aid program since 1977 as a volunteer "victim," instructor, and as past chairman of the First Aid Committee. He trains new instructors for the American Red Cross as well as conducting courses in Advanced First Aid and CPR. Carline developed the curriculum for the Advanced Progression Mountaineering Oriented First Aid Course offered in Seattle, and has taught in many outdoor seminars. He is chairman of The Mountaineers alpine scramblers committee, a program of instruction and non-technical climbing trips, and is a graduate of the Club's basic climbing course. Carline is a member of the faculty of the University of Washington School of Medicine.

INDEX

FIRST AID REPORT FORM

With a sharp knife or razor blade, cut the following four pages out of this book. Tape the pages together to form front and back of the form (see pages 37 and 38 of the book for a reduced scale version), then photocopy the resulting full-size form for your first aid kit.

VITAL SIGN RECORD

Record TIME	BREATHS		PULSE		PULSES BELOW INJURY	PUPILS	SKIN	STATE OF CONSCIOUS-NESS	OTHER
	Rate	Character	Rate	Character					
		Deep, Shallow, Noisy, Labored		Strong, Weak, Regular, Irregular	Strong, Weak, Absent	Equal Size, React To Light, Round	Color, Tempera-ture, Moistness	Alert, Confused, Unresponsive	Pain, Anxiety, Thirst, Etc.

START HERE _____	FINDINGS _____		FIR

AIRWAY, BREATHING, CIRCULATION

INITIAL RAPID CHECK
(Chest Wounds, Severe Bleeding)

ASK WHAT HAPPENED:

ASK WHERE IT HURTS:

TAKE PULSE & RESPIRATIONS	PULSE	RESPIRATIONS

	HEAD: Scalp — Wounds Ears, Nose — Fluid Eyes — Pupils Jaw — Stability Mouth — Wounds	
	NECK: Wounds, Deformity	
	CHEST: Movement, Symmetry	
HEAD-TO-TOE EXAMINATION	ABDOMEN: Wounds, Rigidity	
	PELVIS: Stability	
	EXTREMITIES: Wounds, Deformity Sensation & Movement Pulses Below Injury	
	BACK: Wounds, Deformity	
	SKIN: Color Temperature Moistness	

STATE OF CONSCIOUSNESS

PAIN (Location)

LOOK FOR MEDICAL ID TAG

ALLERGIES

VICTIM'S NAME	AGE
COMPLETED BY	DATE

PORT FORM

T AID GIVEN ——

—————— **RESCUE REQUEST** ——————

Fill Out One Form Per Victim

TIME OF INCIDENT AM PM	DATE

NATURE OF INCIDENT
FALL ON: ☐ ROCK   ☐ SNOW   ☐ FALLING ROCK
☐ CREVASSE   ☐ AVALANCHE
☐ ILLNESS   EXCESSIVE ☐ HEAT ☐ COLD

BRIEF DESCRIPTION OF INCIDENT

INJURIES (List Most Severe First)	FIRST AID GIVEN
SKIN TEMP/COLOR:	
STATE OF CONSCIOUSNESS:	
PAIN (Location):	

TEAR HERE –KEEP THIS SECTION WITH VICTIM

DETACH HERE –SEND OUT WITH REQUEST FOR AID

RECORD:	INITIAL				WHEN LEAVE SCENE
Time					
Pulse					
Respiration					

VICTIM'S NAME		AGE
ADDRESS		
NOTIFY (Name)		

TIME	RELATIONSHIP	PHONE

111

___ SIDE 2 RESCUE REQUEST ___

EXACT LOCATION (Include Marked Map If Possible)

QUADRANGLE: SECTION:

AREA DESCRIPTION:

TERRAIN: □ GLACIER □ SNOW □ ROCK
□ BRUSH □ TIMBER □ TRAIL
□ FLAT □ MODERATE □ STEEP

ON SITE PLANS:
    □ Will Stay Put
    □ Will Evacuate To _____
    Can Stay Overnight Safely □ Yes □ No
    On Site Equipment: □ Tent □ Stove □ Food
    □ Ground Insulation □ Flare □ CB Radio

LOCAL WEATHER

EVACUATION: □ Carry-Out □ Helicopter
    □ Lowering □ Raising

EQUIPMENT: □ Rigid Litter
    □ Food □ Water □ Other

PARTY MEMBERS REMAINING:

____ Beginners ____ Intermediate ____ Experienced

NAME   NOTIFY (Name)   PHONE

NOTIFY:
    IN NATIONAL PARK: Ranger
    OUTSIDE NATIONAL PARK: Sheriff/County Police,
      RCMP (Canada)

TEAR HERE – KEEP THIS SECTION WITH THE VICTIM

DETACH HERE – SEND OUT WITH REQUEST FOR AID